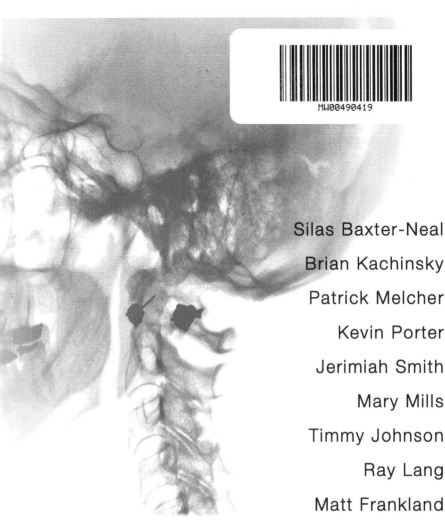

Silas Baxter-Neal

Brian Kachinsky

Patrick Melcher

Kevin Porter

Jerimiah Smith

Mary Mills

Timmy Johnson

Ray Lang

Matt Frankland

Stoyan Angelov

Ariel Ries

TOUGH LIKE YOU

BY AMOS SOMA FULLER

with Greg Bell   Stephanie Person   Krystle Ramos   &   Miriam Zmiewski-Angelova

FIRST EDITION

Library of Congress Cataloging-in-Publication Data (Pending)

p.cm.

Summary: Tough Like You: Injuries, Prevention, Conditioning and Longevity by Amos S. Fuller

ISBN-10: 0-9851148-0-0

ISBN-13: 978-0-9851148-0-0

Fuller, Amos S. (Soma).

Includes references and index.

Copy Editor: Roseanne Segovia

Cover Design: Joey Adamczyk

Tough Like You is available at bulk and wholesale discounts at **sales@toughlikeyou.com**

Contact for Tough Like You at **info@toughlikeyou.com** / **www.toughlikeyou.com**

Thump the World Publishing info@thumptheworldpublishing.com

Printed in the United States of America

Made from eco-friendly, acid-free materials

A percentage of the proceeds from the sale of this book will go toward the health promotion and life skills development for youth via 7G Consultants, LLC.

This book was made possible by generous donations from

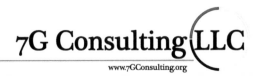

www.7GConsulting.org

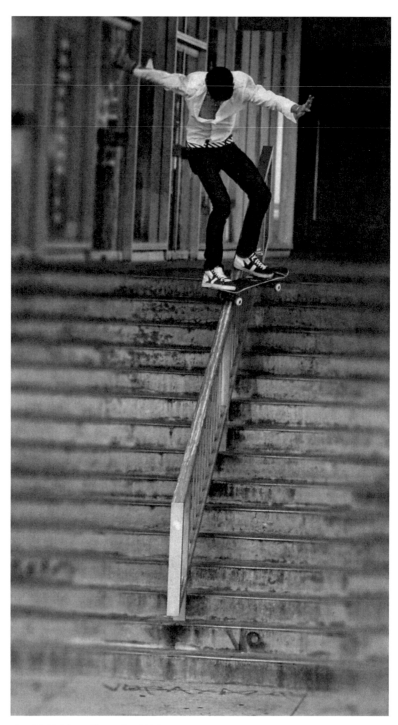

Patrick Melcher   Photo: Seu Trinh

TOUGH LIKE YOU

FOREWORD

FOREWORD

I would love to pitch *Tough Like You* as an answer book, but I have to be honest and not preface it that way. Although the book is filled with preventions, remedies, practical experiences, advice, and solutions to questions you *may* have, it is not designed to answer those questions. *Tough Like You* was written with the fundamental concept of "self-help": the belief that a person can better him or herself by applying the expertise, advice, and experiences of others to their personal needs. In this book, we level the playing field. You will not read about perfect people. They aren't the usual suspects you would find in a book on health. These people are very real. The athletes and health professionals featured are seekers and doers. They feel pain, tire, and experience the same challenges, injuries, mental stressors, and fears that any active person does.

What makes them stand out from the rest is the amazing, almost super human ability to *keep going*. You'll find most of the stories in *Tough Like You* are of people who continue to move forward and progress despite things that would often discourage the average person. Their personal stories, along with a well-rounded wealth of conventional and alternative medical advice, are invaluable. You'll also see some of the most stunning photography, profiling athletes of all ages, shot by highly skilled and dedicated photographers. Action sports photos are simply captivating, no question about it.

People want answers these days and get them faster than any other time in human history. Technology has gifted us with the ability to literally enter a question and instantly receive a list of answers, images, and personal experiences via blogs and websites. It is truly a wonderful thing and is one of the biggest steps people can take to learn more about the world around them. However, I personally believe there is a gap between the knowledge obtained and the knowing of oneself to apply it *usefully*.

Sports, especially action sports (including sports such as gymnastics, martial arts, etc.), force the participant to become seekers in search of what works best for them physically and mentally. That process is exclusively unique to how they train their bodies and mind. Often times through trial and error, the process mimics life itself. Becoming healthier through nontraditional use of the human body, often being prone to risk, is a complex balancing act of "the greater the sacrifice, the greater the reward." As baffling as it may be, it does exist. The X Games first aired on national television a little over a decade ago—a grain of sand in time compared to the history of most sports. Since that time, the perception of action athletes as crazy kids filled with angst has changed to an ever-growing respect of highly skilled individuals that have changed the possibilities of what the human body is capable of doing. Ironically, the majority of them were not drawn to their craft in order to seek any particular results. Unlike jogging, cardio exercises, and many other activities, action artists somewhere and somehow in life found that which instinctually felt like "the right thing to do." There are few action athletes you will find that do it exclusively as a way to stay in shape. Although physical fitness is a by-product of these activities, most are driven— or rather, called— to their passion simply as a developed part of their lifestyle. It becomes who they are, not just *what* they do.

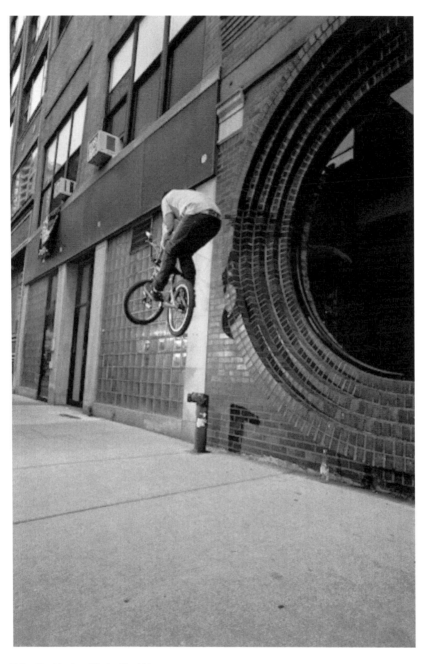

Brian Kachinsky   Photo: David Leep

INTRODUCTION

One of the inspirations for writing this book was sparked by an incident that occurred a few years ago. While skating at Wilson Skate Park in Chicago, located about a yard away from a bike path that spans the entire lakefront, I witnessed a touring cyclist take a bad fall. The intersection near the park is just wrong. Cars exiting a busy Lake Shore Drive have a stop sign at the very same place the bike path crosses the intersection. Cyclists and runners usually play "who's first?" as turning cars and bikes visibly converge. The cyclists move fast. Cars slowly beginning their turn do not notice speeding bikes approaching in time. They either stop or speed up to avoid being an obstacle. Many times the skateboarders and BMX riders at the park hear tires screeching and look toward the corner only to see a car stopped, a bike on the ground, and a person either cursing at the driver or lying on the ground after avoiding a collision. Worst-case scenario: cyclists will slam into the side of the cars. The *very* worst part of this whole intersection is that for years there was coarse gravel that covered the area where the bike path meets the street. It is probably one of the most poorly thought out plans ever.

This particular time, the park was relatively empty but it was still a beautiful, sunny morning. As I was cruising around, I heard that familiar sound "Screeeeeeech!" I looked over and saw a woman on the ground a few feet before the entrance into the street crossing. It was clear that she was cut off, had to brake hard and slid on the gravel to avoid running into the vehicle. The driver had stopped, leaned over her, and asked those famous words heard in my world way too often: "Are you okay?" I knew I had some Band-Aid's and other materials in my bag so I decided to go over.

When I got there, it was obvious from her build, bike, and gear that she rode often. I told her I was skateboarder for years, knew injuries, and asked what was hurt. As I suspected, she had slid on the gravel, lost control of the bike, and got the gift of a nasty knee scrape.

What surprised me was how little she actually knew about what had just happened to her knee. She had some surface damage and I tried to let her know (as tactfully as possible) that she scraped it up pretty badly but it was all skin and she would be all right. She had full mobility of her knee and although it might swell up a bit later, she was basically fine. Her bike suffered no damage. Ironically, those types of skin abrasions really hurt like shit! Skaters and BMX riders know the feeling of losing your palms. There have been times when I have taken large, thick layers off the palms of my hands with gravel embedded too! It really does feel like there's more going on.

During the fall, several pieces of gravel *had* embedded into the surface of her skin. As she called her husband to take her to the hospital, I told her I would clean the wound and apply one of my super cool cloth Band-Aids. I even had some extra large ones that would easily cover her knee wound. She agreed and I rinsed her knee with fresh bottled water while brushing any gravel away. The woman was obviously in pain and would not get up or walk around. I think people have misinterpreted the "don't move the injured" concept. She was determined to go to the hospital which is a perfectly smart thing to do if you really think you need a diagnosis of your injury but a real bummer when you can take a break and ride it out.

The most interesting part of this whole incident was that after I cleaned her knee, she was convinced that there were pebbles in between the skin and her patella. I assured her that there wasn't. I knew that feeling. Falling very hard into the gravel leaves ghost sensations that something is still there. Again, I let her know the gravel didn't find its way next to the bone and was cleaned away. She did not believe me. She insisted there were rocks in her knee and I was not going to argue with her. It was interesting for me to see that she had cycled as a hobbyist for years and still wasn't familiar with her "injured body."

That day was her first step to understanding that pain doesn't always require amputation or even worse, costly emergency room visits only to receive a prescription for Advil.

By the way, I am not a health consultant (they appear later in the book) but I *do* know my place when dealing with other people's bodies. Advice can be offered but again, it's not my body and in no way is the encouragement of "self-healing" a way of discouraging someone from visiting a hospital when they feel it to be necessary. I can only imagine how many times people have suffered from real heart attacks only to be told by those around them, "it's probably just indigestion." Not good. I definitely wouldn't want that on my conscience.

However, I do have some very interesting stories of my self-healing experiences discussed in the forthcoming chapters. One is a long-lasting condition I battled for years. I eventually took action to rid myself of it and was successful. That story even involves sarsaparilla, like they used in the old West tonics. Really.

I believe in a reasonable amount of being your own health care provider. It only makes sense. If being whatever you personally consider healthy to be important, then proactive measures must sometimes be taken.

Health, healing, and longevity are continuous and prevalent driving forces of any living creature on earth. We are inundated with web banners, television commercials, billboards, and interpersonal advice, all on the subject of "what will make you healthier and more alive." Most are not preventative information but "after the fact" quick fixes: lose weight easily, have more energy, the path to clearer skin, the list goes on and on. If you don't believe me, put it to the test. Scan any major browsers or flip through network television stations for five minutes and I guarantee at any time, you will see several of these ads.

From an insect to a Hollywood model, consciously or not, everything we consider life is created with the will, instinct, or autonomic programming to *stay alive*. Resting at the core of that life force will always be the concept of health. Our mental and physical health is *everything*. As the proverbial saying goes, "Without it, we have nothing."

Health is also a very relative concept. It's relative to our personal ideas, surroundings, and pre-existing conditions. It's even relative from species to species. If I was a mosquito that just sucked a belly full of blood on a hot summer day but also had a microscopic tear in my wing that didn't interfere with my ability to fly, I would consider myself healthy. At least instinctually, I would not have the need to medicate or heal. Even though the wing tear would eventually lead to breakage and my death, I would be a happy, 100 percent healthy mosquito until then.

It's much more complicated with us humans. We not only have our instinctive life forces but also thoughts from a complex brain that neuroscientists have only begun to understand. However, like other creatures, we still share the underlying fundamental concept of "no health equals no life."

With that being understood, why do we knowingly do many things that put our health at risk? By necessity, many activities such as driving or flying are an accepted way of life. Conditioned practices like consuming unhealthy foods we were raised on, poor stress-coping skills or crappy sleep habits also affect us. Some are choices that develop into habits, such as smoking, substance abuse, and excessive alcohol usage. There's also a long list of the unhealthy psychological behaviors that help contribute to shortening our chances of leading healthy lives.

These are all questions for a lifetime and definitely *not* ones that will purposely be answered in this book. However, stepping away from these age-old quandaries, we'll take a look at some extraordinary perspectives on what it *does* mean to be healthy. As for longevity, that's another tricky one. Again, here's an area where my focus might differ from the average book on health. Although concerned with living longer and staying healthy forever,

Tough Like You could care less how long you live. It's *how* you live that's important.

Did that sound harsh? What I mean to say is that this body of work is about living *right now*. Fortunately, that right now moves in time and differs for every reader and is always in the present. "Right now" ten years from now is still the present, right? It makes much more sense to condition yourself while doing what you love. Longevity for that reason alone will subsequently better your odds at living longer by default of the conditioning and fortification achieved.

Enough about longevity. It will raise its beautiful gray head in chapters to come anyway. Let's get back to healthy!

We'll take a look at just what *healthy* personally means to the athletes featured in *Tough Like You*. After all, you could live a perfectly healthy life, step outside, and get creamed by a bus today. My take is to learn what works best for you, continue to keep learning more about *your* body and mind, seek help when necessary and *live*.

From the unknowing eye's view, an action athlete is someone who has chosen to go against the instinctual and is often thought of as a having a death wish. They are also sometimes referred to as "thrill seekers." Surely, these must be individuals that for some reason actually *want* to harm themselves or maybe aren't mentally balanced and feel like exceptions to the rules of nature.

Ironically, a member of Deathwish, a skate team with some of the best riders around, was severely injured. Despite that moniker and the perception that they have no regard for their well-being, I can assure you they do care. I personally watched one of their riders heal from a debilitating injury. He eventually went on to perform at his best, subsequently gaining professional status. During the process, the athlete meticulously cared for himself, developing routines and practices that helped him heal. He recovered, rehabilitated, and surpassed his previous best, gracing the covers of several international skate magazines as I wrote this book.

During my days in the Army as a young soldier, I received my requested chance to report to Jump School paratrooper training. I clearly remember hearing friends mouth off the old Army saying: "Only a fool would jump out of a perfectly good airplane." In many ways, it makes sense. It was hilarious to listen to non-Airborne soldiers, or *legs,* joke about an opportunity I felt was an experience that only a fool would pass up. Of course, I didn't feel that way the first few times standing in the door of a C-131 aircraft looking out at the horizon, but that eventually passed. Before every jump, I briefly pondered my mortality. However, I reasoned that the experience of new body movements and unique sensations outweighed the possibility of danger.

After all, how often do we get to do something besides walk, run, or jump up and down? How often do we get to teach our bodies a new way of navigating unusual surroundings like gravity, water, snow, or air?

With total disregard for conventional form, how often do we learn something new that goes beyond our intellect alone?

In the chapters to come, I revisit some of those jumps and how we were taught to fall with three points of body contact to displace the harsh impact of low altitude-to-ground landings. Those techniques became second nature and have stayed with me to this very day.

So if climbing a 2,000 foot rock, skateboarding through traffic, doing handlebar spins on vert, surfing large waves in rough waters, or flying down a snow-covered mountain toward a jump that propels the rider several feet into the air could very well be harmful to our health, *why do we do it*? Again, another question I'm not concerned with, but read on. I'm sure the athletes in later chapters will touch on their personal reasons.

I'm concerned with *how* we do it. We're not talking a racecar with a roll cage flipping twice and the driver walks away. I respect the hell out of NASCAR but I'm concerned with the phenomenon that graced skateboarder Jake Brown when he fell 40 feet, landing with a force several times his body weight. It was a widely televised incident. His shoes popped off from impact and he walked away. It was Jake's body, a few pads, and a hardwood surface. To the general public that accident was "what the fuck just happened" news. It was almost super-human to those that aren't constantly around falls that you can walk away from. Most action athletes just saw it as a gnarly ass fall, with Jake suffering some injuries that would heal. To the average action athlete it was the kind of fall—okay, the kind of *slam*—you would expect on a ramp that size, known as the MegaRamp.

We're going to go deep into the *how*. If you're still stuck on the *why*, by default you'll get that too. Just because one person was quoted as saying, "I climb mountains because they're there," doesn't mean that's why everyone else climbs them. *We all are different*, every single one of us grouped together in a whole world basically doing the same crap but in a billion different ways, each as unique as the patterns on our fingertips. We're all micro-universes within what we call the world, which happens to be in a larger universe. What's beyond all of that, we haven't quite figured out.

I'm a skateboarder, so you'll get a lot of my perspectives as a skateboarder. I'll talk a bit about how I became to be what makes me who I am today. You will read the opinions, advice, and teachings of health care professionals, all of whom stand or have stood in the shoes of an action athlete. There is a treasure chest of stories, straight from the horses' mouths: the athletes themselves.

There are stories of achievements, failures, overcoming, personally learned lessons, and so much more. Professional, amateur, or dedicated hobbyist, you might be surprised to find "tough" doesn't come with a title or acronym besides a name. It's a default badge that sometimes comes with the territory itself.

There's also plenty of jargon that is very specific to the sports and arts that the athletes in the book live for. A helpful glossary of terms is located in the back for quick reference. A "sex-change" in *Tough Like You* would not be a medical procedure but rather a body position. That didn't sound right either. Just check the glossary when confused.

Concepts like *health* or *healthy* will take on a whole new meaning from the eyes of an action athlete. As a skateboarder, if I tell you "I'm healthy," that means "It's on." "Let's skate." "Where you at fool, meet me at the spot!"

I could have a tumor the size of an orange bulging out of my neck but "healthy" in our language means "able to skate." The rat hole goes even deeper, having various understood degrees of "healthy." If I'm at 50 percent, that means, "Yeah, I'm cruising with you but don't expect any hammers or attempts." I can skate, but I'm not primed. When an action athlete is at 100 percent, it's known. They glow like a mid-July Chicago sky. There is nothing better than the feeling of not feeling anything that inhibits or distracts. We'll get more into that later. I must emphasize that the aforementioned conversations on health are frequent among action athletes and take place more than people could ever imagine.

For a bunch of perceived reckless, thrill-seeking death wishers with no concern for their well being, skaters, bikers, climbers, surfers, and other action athletes sure do talk a heap about being, or not being, healthy. *Who would've thought?*

Brandon Cole   Photo: Larry LaMar

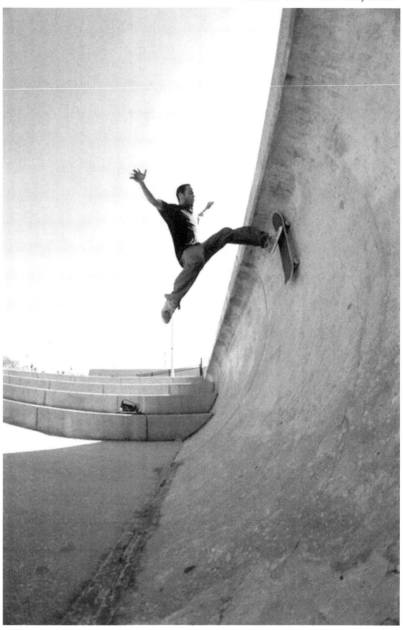

In this chapter, we'll talk a bit about expanding and contracting. This was a land. Brandon Cole rolled away— probably one of the furthest body extensions a skater has done without ever actually leaving the board. Even a Christ Air has a little more flesh on the board. Nice.

1

"Everyone says it's about getting back up. I say it's what you do when you get up that's important and when you find yourself doing it again, you'll be that much better at getting up when you're really down."

—Koji Kraft

FALLING DOWN

If not for the fear of a class action lawsuit, I would ask all my readers to slowly lower themselves halfway to the floor…and fall. You might be surprised to find it actually wasn't that bad. Falling is the one of the few activities we all practiced at some point in our lives. From toddler to teen, we became masters at the art of falling. Sometimes graceful, other times faint and dramatic, often clumsy and rarely stealth ninja-like. We all spent years picking ourselves up from the ground. Gravity has a funny way of bringing unsupported matter down to earth.

It's funny that the history of entertainment has always used tripping, falls, and shoves as the core attention-grabber in not only comedies like *The Three Stooges* but also in westerns and thrillers. In a good western, it isn't the punch or gunshot that catches your attention but rather the fall after the gunshot that creates the scene. Nowadays there are reality shows that pop up out of nowhere, with home video entries of mishaps and sports blunders, and even shows with contestants that compete to navigate courses without falling. The ending highlights of these shows always features clips of the funniest or scariest falls. For a society obsessed with watching people fall down or off of things, we sure are very sensitive about falling in real life.

Maybe it has to do with the perception that after a certain age, it is no longer acceptable and cheapens our dignity. The funny thing is, we all stumble, miss a step, stub toes, slip on ice, and more. Public figures under camera scrutiny are recorded missing a step or falling during a performance more often than most.

With all that being said and with us all having experienced falling through our formative years, why do we suck at it so badly later in life? Loss of primal instinct? We walk upright and once we learned how to strut, there's usually no looking back. Think about it: animals don't fall often, but they are *incredible* at falling. They lose balance, run into each other, misstep, or fall, and instantly go into "self-correcting" mode. Turtles might be the exception; they have it kind of rough and don't recover from being flipped so easily.

Have you ever really thought about the skill it takes for a full-grown horse to fall at a high speed and adjust their bodies back to running? It's simply *amazing* to think that the same horse would have to go through hours of training to perform far less complex human taught "tricks," but can recover from a fall that it learned naturally during early development.

I'm a firm believer that like all animals and mammals—oh wait, we are mammals; we just drive cars and have iPads—we literally unlearn our ability to tuck, roll, bend, balance, fall, and recover as we age.

We're not apples! Why do some of us just drop like a damn piece of fruit from a tree? I think that Fig Newton, Isaac Hayes dude needs to help us out here.

Action athletes are most certainly the honey crisp apples of the bunch. We float down off the branch, roll around a few times, and pop into your hands yelling, "Bite me!" At worst, we obey Newton's law, slam into the ground, bruise ourselves, and have a buddy put us in the basket. Either way, we're usually edible after a while, bad apples of the bunch or not.

BIG YOU, LITTLE ME

I remember buying my son one of those expanding plastic gadgets made of short plastic connectors for the holidays. That thing was the shit! I was amazed at how this dense web of colorful plastic rods could go from a soccer ball shape and size to a perfect circle several times larger, hollow and firm. I would always randomly pick it up and expand, contract, expand, contract—that's pretty much all you could do with it. You definitely need a child's imagination to push that thing any further. I could see it being a damn good planet, prison, or force field if I was still a tyke. However, when I decided to write a full body of work concerning what skateboarding has taught me in relation to health, that toy reminded me of our bodies, or vice versa.

We usually occupy a lot more space than we realize, and while at the same time we have the ability to selectively shrink ourselves to a fraction of that occupied space. I also will never forget seeing some yogi on a late night show stuffing himself in a little clear cube, both awesome and yucky at the same time—awesome as hell that it was real and not an illusion, and *yuck* that the freakin' box was clear. That was borderline pornographic. No one should ever have to see a box-o-skin! But I thank the dude from the bottom of my heart for being that skilled and exposing me to what later in life would be the first of learning my untapped physical and psychological potentials. Skin and glass: ugh.

Few will ever attain such flexibility, but we (action athletes) have become quite good at using our amazing shrinking abilities to survive bails. For the record, a bail is getting out and away from a missed attempt and a fall is, well, a fall. However, we do have several names to describe what kind of fall it is and how severe.

Just about all of us, at all times, take up anywhere from 6.5 to 9 feet. If we were to hamster-ball ourselves, we would need some large spheres in order to stretch our arms and spread our legs even 45 degrees in relation to circumference. At the same time, almost all of us can fit in a box a fourth the size of what that giant hamster ball would be. Yes, weight, mass, and straight out fat does matter, but overall, it's possible.

My photographer friend and I did a little shoot to illustrate the difference in space we took up stretched out da Vinci Vitruvian Man style and then compressed fetal-like. More than the common knowledge of "yes, we can curl up and be smaller" was the actual measurements that proved interesting. Personally, I wanted to construct human-fitting hamster balls to illustrate the point but it just wasn't in the budget.

This expanding and contracting is a daily way of life for us from full-out to full-in and all in between.

5' 3"

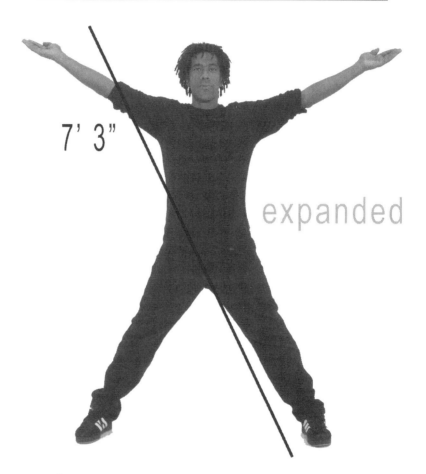

7' 3"

expanded

Soma Age: 44 Height: 6'1" Weight: 195lbs

compressed

2' 8"

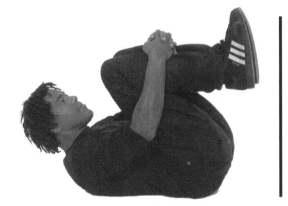

2' 6"

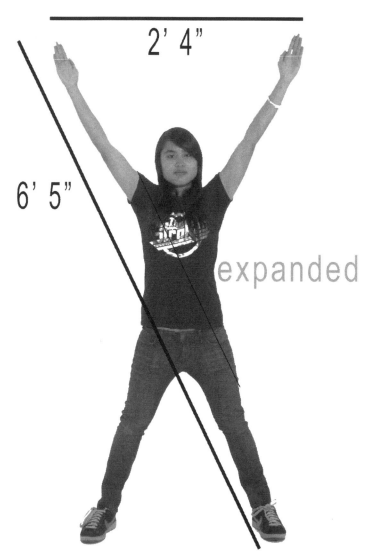

2' 4"

6' 5"

expanded

Amy Age: 21 Height: 5'1" Weight: 105lbs

compressed

2' 4"

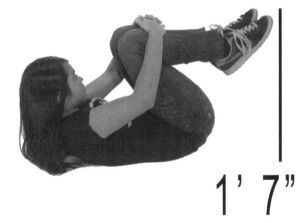

1' 7"

As you can see, the numbers differ tremendously. Bailing a trick from an attempted Frontside Crook that was sticky would usually involve running midair, with arms flailing (extended) to stop or fall. During that bail, a person could easily cover over 20 feet of total area and distance depending on speed. So why the hell is this even important? It's important to know what's around you and how close in proximity. Are you in a park with several people around, or speeding down a run between trees and other natural obstacles? Or better yet, a tight street spot surrounded by metal, concrete, and moving vehicles?

In comparison, many other falls involve instantaneous ground or floor contact. Depending on the speed in which traveling, these are almost always "tuck and roll" situations. Action athletes are accustomed to compressing themselves into a form that will literally make them roll. Using this during forward momentum to ground impact *greatly* lessens the chance of injury. Note: I said injury! Tuck and rolls still usually leave you pretty sore, especially after a good number of them in one session. Sleep it off.

STAND IN THE DOOR

"Anyone in the Airborne community can relate to the famous phrase, 'Any time you walk away from a jump, it's a good jump.' Sometimes, however, soldiers don't walk away—they either limp or are carried from the drop zone. Accidents during Airborne operations are common, ranging from a weak or improper parachute landing fall (PLF) to soldiers misjudging clearance of ground objects. Airborne operations are unforgiving!"

As an action athlete *and* former paratrooper, I know that learning to fall from military jumps has helped me with my ability to fall without serious injury. The similarities between the two are more than comparable. In jump school, we learned to fall with three points of contact moving at a 45 degree angle: first on the buttocks, then rolling to the fatty area of the thigh, then resting to the side of the lower legs. Most falls in action sports end up playing out a version of this technique as discussed before. Breakdancing is probably the ultimate conditioning for falls. Bust out the linoleum!

Be it skating, biking, snowboarding, or climbing, we all stand in the door and jump on a regular basis. Whether we walk away or don't has to do with many factors. It's good to have the ability to control the factors that we can because there is a plethora of things that we can't.

SLAMMED

In case of emergency, your fingers, hips, shoulders, head, toes, knees, elbows, heels, and tailbone *can* be used as a cushioning device. It's just gonna hurt like hell and you might not walk away!

The truth is that these are only the basics when teaching someone how to fall. It's a hands-on experience. There are definite no-no's and good advice like, "Never just put your hands down to take full impact and hope for the best." Statistically, the number one action sports injury is a fractured wrist or broken arm. That's because our initial reaction when falling is to break the fall with our hands. Over time and with more experience in bailing or falling situations, we learn to make our fingers and hands the first point of contact, helping to reposition our bodies for what's coming. In a fraction of a second, hands and fingers touch the surface, release, and guide the rest of the body from the blow of the full, initial force.

Many times, injury is imminent. Sessions are full of swellbows, hippers, ankle tweaks, and others. Most of those, however, are not session stoppers. Knowing how to fall increases an athlete's confidence when trying to learn something new. Preferably, not falling would be the best situation. Good luck.

I fell from a 13 foot vert ramp before, from *lip* (see glossary) to flat. Somehow my body positioned itself midair to fall in a sideways fetal position. It was at Scrap, an indoor bike park in Hoffman Estates, Illinois. The park was inside a multi-sports arena with soccer fields and ice hockey. After the fall, I walked away or at least got up. I was told the sound was so loud, it was heard in the soccer fields yards away—and I had a helmet on. When I hit the flat I immediately stood up and started looking for my glasses that would easily blend into the wood grain tone and get crushed. As I looked for my glasses, the people on the deck were yelling for me to sit down. I thought to myself, "Why?" I yelled back to them, "Hey, I'm looking for my glasses!" They kept yelling gibberish until I finally realized part of that gibberish was "Your glasses are on your face dude, SIT DOWN!"

Although I felt okay and was used to popping up after falls, I was stunned. The helmet not only saved my head but its snug fit kept my glasses from coming off. Imagine seeing some dumbass fall 13 feet, get up, and wander aimlessly around the bottom of a one story high ramp. My elbows and hips were badly bruised. It hurt for days but eventually healed.

If any of my limbs would have been extended and hit first, they would've most certainly broken on impact.

I don't wear a helmet every time I hop on my board but I will always assess a situation now for potential danger and gear up appropriately. A vert ramp is always an appropriate "gear up" time. For any beginner action sports enthusiast, a helmet is just plain smart. After a while, you can decide whether or not to risk the potential chance of a head injury.

That might not exactly be a politically correct opinion but it *is* the reality for 90 percent of action athletes. Once an advanced skill level is met, many only use helmets when trying something new, riding big, or when required by public facilities that mandate wearing head protection, and rightfully so. Knee and elbow protection is also strongly encouraged or required by many facilities. Sorry hips; no protection out there for you. It's contusion cloud nine and hipper heaven!

There are plenty of stories about falls from the featured athletes in *Tough Like You*. As you will find in chapters to come, diet, flexibility, conditioning, experience, and more play an essential role in the techniques you personally develop for your particular style of being as tough as you can be. All in all, slams, bails, and falls don't have to be and usually aren't catastrophes.

Any active person should constantly access their limitations, environment, physical condition, equipment, and state of mind. All these contribute to how you perform and if you're ready to push your limits...or not.

Corey Hendricks   Photo: Lee Larkins

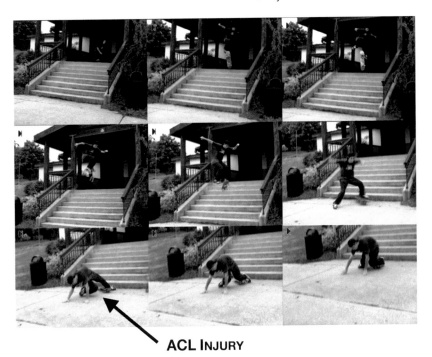

ACL INJURY

Corey Hendricks is one of the best skateboarders around. I don't feel bad using his past ACL injury as an example. It fact, it's the only visual of a photographed injury in *Tough Like You*.

There are plenty of worded descriptions by the athletes themselves but this isn't a reality show type of book that glorifies gore and injury. These aren't goofs trying to impress someone by doing something they aren't capable of doing.

This photo is a documentation of a good athlete taking a bad fall. **Action Sports are dangerous and injuries do happen. If you go into it knowing that, you'll survive.**

As mentioned in the chapter "Falling Down," you'll notice that Corey's body went from being fully extended to being very compressed. The speed, distance, and height combined with an *unfortunate* angle, caused injury. This was one of the times he wasn't able to walk away, despite having stuck it several times before. Skateboarding is funny like that.

Like Corey, the next chapter contains very skilled athletes that have experienced bad injuries and healed. You'll notice ACL mentioned quite a bit. It is a very vulnerable area for the maneuvers we execute.

2

"I won't quit skating until I am physically unable."

—Tony Hawk

YOU OKAY?

I'd like to introduce you to some extraordinary athletes and artists. Straight from the proverbial horses' mouths, in their own words, you'll find their stories to have similarities to your own experiences. There's no particular order in which they are featured; no ranking system here. They range from pros, amateurs, legends, rippers, and unknowns. Carefully selected, they are winners. All practitioners in the "art of living," they span the spectrum of age, gender, and experience with personal and unique reasons for being as tough as they are.

My first experience watching Silas skate in person was at a local park. He and a friend were having a blast doing the craziest high-speed nose grinds across a short box. Grinding as if the lip truly had butter on it, both would pop out with more speed than they started with and continued to ravage the park "follow the leader" style. They were just goofing off, but I was watching an impromptu demo from one of the best.

A few weeks later and after a few conversations, I remember Silas mentioning he was eager to repair a fence at home but was bummed it would have to wait due to his travel plans. He was that kind of guy, seriously down to earth. Ironically, after not seeing him around for a while, I was flipping through *Skateboarder Magazine* and read the "Skate Anatomy" interview where he described slicing his finger almost to the bone while building a fence for his garden. It's not easy being green...or really good if ya think about it.

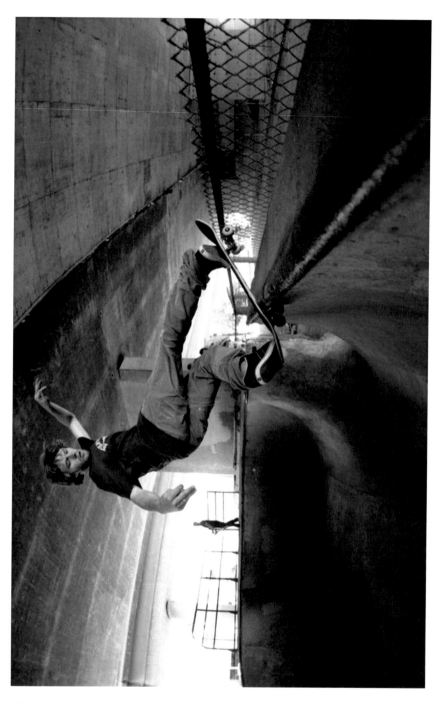

Photo: Courtesy of Silas Baxter-Neal & *Racket Magazine*

SILAS BAXTER-NEAL

"You fuck around, you lay around." —Kerry Getz

29

PROFESSIONAL SKATEBOARDER

18 YEARS SKATING

HOMETOWN: EUGENE, OR

CURRENT LOCATION: PORTLAND, OR

At the age of 16, I broke three bones in my foot, was in a cast for five months, and off my board for seven months. Two months after I started skating again, I broke my arm and had a full cast up to my shoulder for five months. I've also had several ankle sprains, ligament damage, and a hernia that eventually healed.

I rarely participate in skateboard contests, but every now and again I check them out and see people I wouldn't see otherwise. At one particular contest, I was skating around during "practice" and rolled my ankle pretty severely. I went to the hospital, got X-rays, and was checked out to make sure it wasn't more serious than a sprain because it felt much worse. They said I had ligament damage and told me to stay off of it. It sounded easy except for the fact that I was scheduled to leave two days later for a three week skating camping trip in Europe that I had been looking forward to for months.

On this trip I didn't skate, but I didn't stay off my foot either. Instead, I hobbled around from spot to spot trying not to be left behind. **That was the beginning of a series of re-occurring ankle injuries that lasted for two years**.

After that trip, I went home to Chicago and did my best to stay off the ankle, but as soon as it felt good enough to ride around on, I would schedule myself on another skate trip. Usually I was able to skate during the first few days, but I would always end up injuring my ankle again whether it was another roll from loose ligaments or just me wearing it out. I followed this routine for about a year: resting at home for 2–3 weeks then on to another skate trip for two weeks and came home limping every time. Eventually, I started to favor the other ankle so much that I ended up rolling and injuring that one as well.

At this point, I decided that I needed some outside help to get better. I started seeing two physical therapists (Dr. Joseph, formerly from Advanced Physical Medicine located in Hoffman Estates, IL and Dr. Gee). They determined that not only had I damaged the ligaments, but had also bruised the bones in the socket between my ankle and my leg bone. Because of this bruising, the whole joint was swollen, causing the ligament to stay stretched and ultimately getting less stretchy and more brittle. They put me on an exercise routine that strengthened not just my ankle but also my legs, core, and back. The routines were very simple in nature and through repeating the same simple movements, the rest of my body was helped by taking the extra burden off my injured ankles, allowing them to heal and eventually strengthen.

One thing that I found unique about these two doctors was that they were very interested in the movements I did when I skated and had me skate around the parking lot so they could see how my body moved and what muscle groups they needed to work on. After about a year of physical therapy (and finally taking two months off the board), my ankles made a serious recovery and they function close to how they used to.

I learned more about how well the body is connected and how all your muscles work together to help each other—the arm bone is connected to the hand bone, or however that song goes…

Now I try to practice the obvious: stretch before you do anything that exerts your muscles, eat good food, don't drink too much, yada, yada, yada. As simple as that seems, it's actually hard to follow.

I believe my experiences with injuries and healing has helped me be more conscious of what I am doing with my body and whether it's helpful or not.

Injuries are hard to prevent. They happen when they happen; no one *tries* to get hurt. What we do is reckless in nature and so therefore, injury is almost inevitable.

I now know that not resting while injured can do more damage then the initial injury itself. As maddening as it is, the best thing to do when you get hurt is to chill.

About one third into writing this complete body of work, I received an unexpected email from Brian Kachinsky asking me to tell him more about this *Tough Like You* book project. Surprised and frankly honored, I did. It only took a few exchanges before Brian agreed to be a featured athlete. That week, the BMX and skate gods aligned with the stars, moon, and sun. That week was pretty fucking good. Brian does things on a bike that look physically impossible to me. Prior to us discussing the book, I found myself in his private indoor bike park, "The Bakery," moving some ramps. Everything was big, steep, and scary. BMX takes some heart.

"Kachinsky, the clean-cut Midwesterner with a pleasant demeanor and a limitless supply of corny jokes, takes on a different persona when it comes to attacking daunting handrails all over the world. With the focus of a prizefighter engaged in the bout of his life, he doesn't quit until he gets what he wants, taking repeated slams if necessary. He's made the top 5 in each of his three X Games Street appearances, topping out with bronze in 2010. With a style that's equal parts tech and manly, he likes to use the entire course and tries to deliver something unique whenever possible."

—Brian Tunney, ESPN.com

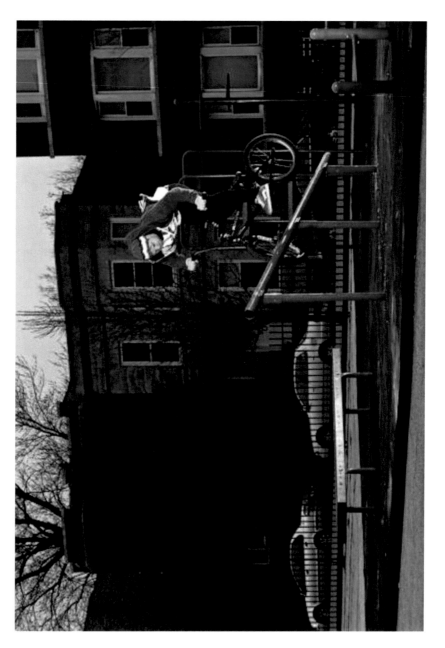

Brian Kachinsky   Photo: David Leep

BRIAN KACHINSKY

"A ship in the harbor is safe, but that's not what ships are for."

—John A. Shedd

29

PROFESSIONAL BMX

17 YEARS RIDING

HOMETOWN: NEENAH, WI

CURRENT LOCATION: CHICAGO, IL

I'm currently recovering from my third career ACL reconstruction. I have fake teeth, some shoulder issues, back issues, etc. but all in all I'm pretty healthy.

I eat mostly fresh foods, avoid fast food, and only drink on occasion. Diet, exercise, and perseverance have been the keys to my success.

I feel like I've had it all at some point: broken bones, fake teeth, surgeries, degenerative discs, rotator cuff issues, tons of stitches and have been to emergency rooms in more than eight countries including Germany, Mexico, Netherlands, Thailand, China, Estonia, and Brazil. I've worked with countless physical therapists, both standard and holistic. I have also gained a good amount of knowledge on the human body and how it works and heals in the process.

I got invited to the first big tour of my career in 2002 and was obviously excited. On the first day of the tour I was on fire, pulling everything I tried until I got carried away. I fell on a big gap-to-rail manual at Chenga 2, a skate park in Cleveland, Ohio and tore my ACL. I finished the tour and even rode a bit on the last day despite my knee being a mess. I ended up getting surgery (a patella tendon graft) and was on the road to recovery for the next six months. I learned during this period that no matter how messed up one part of your body is, you can still work other parts of your body. My arms, shoulders, core, and the rest of my body got so strong during this rehab process. Despite attending the biggest party school in the nation at the time (UW Madison), I often avoided alcohol and drugs as I knew it would not help my healing. To each their own, but I was so driven to get back that I didn't want anything to delay that progress. I was determined to come back stronger than before. I succeeded and ended up having a great year the following year. **Hard work pays off.**

I have many more stories but that's the first major one that I recall. One crazy story includes taking an emergency flight back from China to get my leg drained after three Chinese hospitals wouldn't do it. I've also gotten stitches using twine in Estonia with no anesthetic. The list goes on and on.

I think so much of it is mental. I think your mental state and pain tolerance has a lot to do with it. Motivation is also a huge factor. It's easy to forget how awesome it feels to ride and skate when you've been out for a while. **You need to constantly remind yourself how awesome it feels to ride and use that as your motivation while you are healing and rehabilitating**.

I have learned from every single injury I've ever had and each has taught me about the body and how to hopefully avoid that injury in the future or at least better care for it if it does happen again.

I eat a balanced diet of unprocessed foods—lots of greens and anything with anti-inflammatory properties. I also eat some lean meats and lots of grains and fiber. Water is the most important. I drink a ton of water. I also drink black coffee which I should probably cut back on, but I think it's fine in moderation as well. I drink from time to time but not daily and only in social situations. I also take a multivitamin, calcium, and fish oil for various reasons. All of these are a way of life. My diet isn't super strict because I feel that it can sometimes result in overeating but I'd say I have a pretty sensible diet. I stretch before I ride and try to always "warm up" a bit if I have the chance. I have also done yoga in the past but don't on a regular basis. Hopefully that changes soon.

Style, artistic creativity, longevity, and personality might sound like some marketing review to you, but I can't think of any other way to write it. Patrick's name actually preceded him in my life as a skateboarder. I heard the name tossed around long before meeting and sharing a skate spot with him.

My first experience watching him skate was the shit and a bag of chips. The dude definitely has his *own* style. It's multidimensional, using his whole body, physiology, natural elements, and other structures when skating.

Melcher is a survivor. He survived the short-sighted business world of skateboarding and corporate crap, the physical world of putting his body through decades of hard work, and most of all, the challenge of being himself.

Most legends don't like the label, so I'll shut up. No label needed though, because beyond legacy, Patrick is *still* creating. On or off the board, from interviews with *GQ* to recently holding the official title of "second-best moustache in the world," the dude is an artist to be respected.

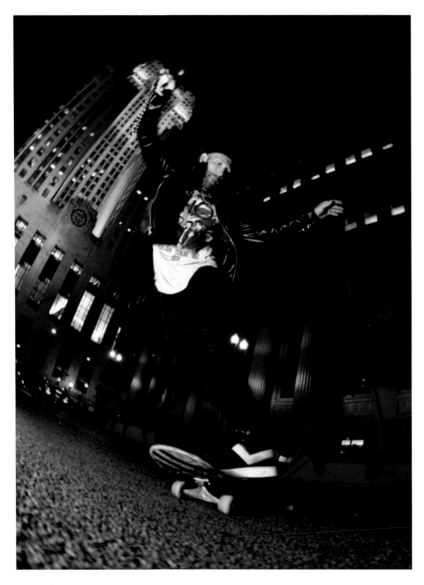

Photo: Courtesy of Patrick Melcher

PATRICK MELCHER

"If you're going through hell, keep going."

—Winston Churchill

34

LEGENDARY SKATEBOARDER

OVER 20 YEARS SKATING

HOMETOWN: ROCKFORD, IL

CURRENT LOCATION: LOS ANGELES, CA

While growing up in Northern Illinois, I learned to use what environment I had to make the best of a good time wherever I was. This usually included causing mischief and some sort of activity. Always making it about the fun that we were having, skateboarding soon took over my life and became the driving force behind almost every action.

One pivotal moment in my adolescence was when my local skate park had a disaster: the roof caved in due to massive snow build-up. The skate park, where I had come of age athletically, was in ruins and no longer useable. I joined forces with a couple of other skateboarders and a BMX rider and in 1994, we decided to build our own private terrain.

The PIT (private indoor terrain) lasted for 10 years. Having 24-hour access to a skate park that I had a large hand in designing really helped to launch my ambition into the realm of professionalism. Taking initiative by getting the skate park going and maintaining it over time gave me a real "do it yourself" (DIY) sense of personal action which I transferred over into various other sections of my life.

A second turning point came when I made the move from the Midwest out to California. Meeting my skate heroes and hooking up with all the industry heads was exactly what I needed at the time. **I got sponsored, filmed a video part, and was ready to turn pro when I inevitably shattered my right knee**. It was a disastrous setback, tearing all the ligaments in my knee, and it took a lot of therapy and time to get back into working order.

A couple of years after that I found myself ripping better than ever and turned pro for my favorite team. Eight years deep into my pro skateboarding career, I find myself living in Los Angeles and still shredding.

At the time of this interview I feel relatively healthy. All parts are up and running. No complaints.

Here's a breakdown of some of my past injuries: I've had a broken shoulder, which required one month in traction plus six more weeks in a braced shoulder-splinted cast attached to my hip (It was a nightmare.). I've broken all of my fingers. Yes, all of them—the left pinky six times. I've ruptured my left testicle. It's just mush now, all veins and mushy stuff, but the right one works okay so I can still have kids. I've broken each elbow twice, broken my left ankle, and my left big toe.

When you are amped on your sport, you live for it. The thing that happened with my knee was physically disastrous. It was in the late '90s when it seemed that jumping down bigger and bigger obstacles was the status quo. I was attempting a 180 down a big ass set of stairs. I had already pulled it once but wasn't totally satisfied with my roll away; it looked a little sketchy on the video playback. So I said the famous last words: "One more try." Something went wrong and upon impact I folded my leg sideways.

I instantly knew it was fucked. I came down from an 18-stair free fall and landed on all of my weight, snapping my knee inward; it was a blazing shock to the system. As I lay on the ground, I tried to straighten my knee out and heard and felt all kinds of popping and crunching. This was mad scary. I instantly thought to myself, "I fucking tore my ACL, I know it!"

Agony set in as the homies helped me get to the ER. An MRI revealed the gnarly truth: a torn ACL, MCL, and medial meniscus. First, the doctor did an arthroscopic sweep to try and clear out the shattered cartilage and repair the MCL. After that, I went to rehab to get back into a better muscular condition to prepare for surgery.

This all took time, which I was particularly bummed about. I just wanted them to go in and fix everything at once. They had to do three surgeries and insisted that I do therapy between each one which would suck up three weeks each time. Fuck that. All I wanted was to get back on the board.

The second surgery was the major one. Then they had to open up my knee and replace the ACL. The three surgeries and six months of physical therapy would leave me scarred physically as well as mentally. I knew that this injury was the big one. I had heard about various other pros having this same injury and what a toll it takes on a person. It was 1998 and using synthetic ligaments wasn't all that popular yet. I needed a new ACL and the whole cadaver thing wasn't an option either. So the doctor removed a ligament from my upper thigh and fabricated a new ACL out of it.

The third surgery came when my knee didn't seem to be attached correctly and there was still a piece of cartilage floating underneath my kneecap. It caused my knee to lock into a straight position and was seriously painful. They scoped it again and cleared all of it up.

Up to the point when I had the injury, the way I was living my life was 24/7 skateboarding. It was eat, drink, sleep skateboarding, 100 percent, all the time. When the knee injury happened, it felt like I had my whole life stripped out from under me. My passion, my heart, all gone. This is the part where I learned that focusing all of your passion on one endeavor is a volatile thing.

Without skateboarding, I felt really lost. I was 20 years old and looking at a long and painful recovery. Every friend I had, I'd met through skating. All the music I liked had come one way or another through skating too. My ethos on life, my likes and dislikes, all stemmed from skating. Without this activity I wouldn't be anything, and now I had no real passion. I didn't want to read the magazines or watch the videos anymore. I knew the itch would be too fucked for me to handle, kind of the same way I hate going to watch contests that I am not skating in. If I'm just looking on and not able to skate the obstacles, I get all tense and freaked out.

I put it all behind me. I was a sponsored am (amateur) getting ready to go pro, had a career-affecting injury, and now had to re-evaluate my path—tough stuff for an adolescent. But we are skateboarders; we are fucking tough. **I kept thinking of all the dudes who had been through this thing already; dudes like Danny Way (my hero). I actually looked to football player Jerry Rice for inspiration.**

Now, I'm not a football fan by any means, but it just so happens that Jerry Rice blew out his knee the same week I did. The dude came back in like four weeks and was back on the field in NFL games. If he can do it, I can skate again, no problem.

I dove into school and found a ton of other stuff to focus on like therapy, bike riding, chess, and lots of reading. When I was ready to skate again, I started off softly. I skated when I wanted and tried to focus on school. This was a life-changing injury in more ways than one. Not only did it stifle my pro career, but it taught me to moderate my focus on singular activities. I thought, there's no way I'm making skating my WHOLE life again just to have it stripped away for a second time. This is the part of my life where I figured out that skating is fun and I'm just gonna have fun with it.

That is where I have been ever since. This simple philosophy of not taking it too seriously let me develop in the natural way that I feel I was meant to all along. Every time I'm on my board, I let the enjoyment of skating guide me. If it gets frustrating and not fun, I recognize that and stop.

I've been straight edge my whole life. I've never had a drink, never smoked, and have never taken any medicine that wasn't administered by a doctor. **I let my body heal itself as best as it can**. I realize this is not a very conventional way to live, but it's what works for me.

I eat food when I'm hungry. That's it. Nothing preachy. I go out to bars a lot (five times a week) but I just don't indulge. I want people to party and have fun and I don't judge anybody else for what they do. I'm actually pretty impressed with the party guy lifestyle when those guys can pull off a gnarly career of heavy athletics. I guess that's why most of my homies are pretty heavy ragers.

Due to Kevin's heavy schedule, we decided to wait a bit and have a nice, quiet sit down at my place while he was in town for the holidays. I hadn't seen KP in months and was eager to get his story. I knew it was good. He has always been a good vibe guy, one of those people that no matter what is going on in life, he has something positive to say. I think Kevin and I had actually become friends by default, as mediators at Wilson Skate Park where bikes technically were not allowed. Occasionally because of the difference in lines bikes and skaters took, an argument would break out. Most skaters didn't mind bikes and the bikers that were conscious knew how to ride without interference anyway. It was usually the guy with a chip on his shoulder, be it skater or biker, who would start some crap. There were several times when we would try to be the voice of reason and ease tension.

It was refreshing to have a conversation *away* from the park. So with coffee in hand, KP spilled his guts about his life on a bike frame which includes him kinda literally spilling his guts and what makes him who he is today.

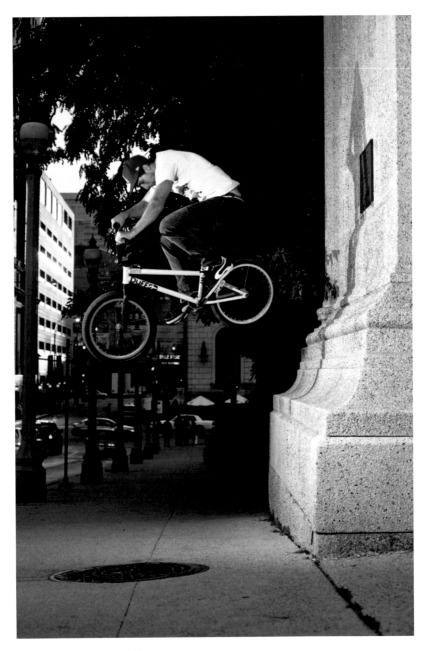

Kevin Porter   Photo: David Leep

KEVIN PORTER

"When something bad happens, something good always comes out of it." — Self Quote

29

PROFESSIONAL BMX

20 YEARS RIDING

HOMETOWN: BURBANK, IL

CURRENT LOCATION: LONG BEACH, CA

A bike rider for 20 years, I've been riding since I was nine. I'm a compassionate person and believe in equality for everybody. That usually translates into my bike riding because riding is a performance art. I'm not someone that likes to compete, although I am in competition for industry purposes. **I like to find things that people don't regularly do, throw it out there, and see what happens in return**.

Man, I've got a laundry list of past injuries—20 years of bike riding will do that to you. My major injuries: I had my toes pinned. I had knee surgery at the age of 24. (It was a scope; not reconstructive at all.) It was a bursitis that needed to be cleaned which resulted in a two-year recovery because I wasn't conscious about the recovery; I was just doing it and did it improperly and I didn't follow instructions. I was young and just behaved poorly. It was a very simple procedure that I mistreated and it caused years of recovery. Other than that, I've had a lot of rolled ankles, probably each ankle twice. I've had two broken big toes that, again, I didn't allow to heal properly. I have serious bunion problems which I go to yoga every day to try and heal without surgery. I have a massaging piece at my house that I work on. It's seriously going to be a seven year process massaging that thing out which is terrible because it could have taken me two months to fix. My biggest injury was when I lost my spleen at the age of 22.

My spleen injury started when I was 15. I had been diagnosed with mononucleosis, which is pretty common. My spleen was enlarged at that point. I spent three weeks healing, did exactly what the doctor said, and it shrunk. But from that time until the time I was 22, it never really shrunk to the size that it needed to.

When I was 22, I was drinking a lot and was very unhealthy. I was a vegetarian but I didn't have the good nutritional understanding I needed. I was in the worst shape of my life. I remember being at a contest; I was riding across a handrail, fell off, and fell flat onto my stomach. My whole body hit the ground like a pancake. It was very abrupt but it didn't hurt. It was like, "Wow. That was weird." What I assume happened was that I enlarged my spleen. I knew I re-injured it because for the next couple of months I was lethargic.

I didn't go to the doctor; I didn't feel like I necessarily needed to. I thought I was just eating improperly or drinking too much.

I went on a mega-tour trip just for props. For some odd reason I was experimenting with chewing tobacco and became addicted which is so bad because I was putting metals and all sorts of things into my body. You can imagine how torn and beat up my body was, trying to recuperate the whole time but never did. You need to be on a light diet with a spleen injury like that, and let your body take all the time it needs to bring it back to its normal shape. Anyway, I did a simple trick, landed on my stomach, and kind of punched myself which exploded my spleen. It was so uncomfortable. I was lying in every position. Normally, I get hurt a lot and can usually sit in one position and breathe it out and assess the situation, but this situation was not going anywhere. I said to myself, "Man, this is ridiculous." **I went to the hospital and the next thing I knew I woke up and I had no spleen!**

I spent two weeks in the hospital. I was on IVs and all that stuff. It was so bad, but they did what they had to do. They took my spleen out and I had a stitching surgery that was a brand new process where they stitched my muscle back together and glued my skin so that the scar wouldn't look as big on my stomach but inside I had a big, bulky knot.

I spent a month totally careless about the injury. I thought, "Hey my spleen is gone. I don't have to worry about it." I just thought I needed the cut to heal up properly. About a month and a half later, a little after my 22nd birthday, I was vomiting profusely. I could not stop vomiting. Vomit, vomit, vomit. It went on for 24 hours. I thought I had the flu. What actually happened was that the surgery they gave me caused a bowel blockage. I was in the hospital for another two weeks. Basically, the scar tissue was pushing up against one of my bowels, not allowing anything to pass. The bowel blockage occurred because that injury and my skin should have been more relaxed. Every movement that I made that month caused calcium deposit to build up on the back of my skin and created a scar in my stomach that could have been a lot smaller. Again, this was another unconscious healing process that I took. People don't understand that just eating in general takes energy away from your body. If you eat a big hunk of food, your body has to do its job to recover. I'm 29 now and in that time I've thought about all these injuries and all these things that I've done. If I knew what I know today back then, my situation could be totally different.

On top of the spleen injury, just falling and losing my spleen and going through that pain for so long made me lose the ability to be the rider that I wanted to be. I couldn't reach those points where I could be completely comfortable on my bike and want to ride because I always had that injury at the back of my head. And this goes along with my knee. Exactly the same deal with my knee.

I learned that I lost half of my immune system that day. It was such a detrimental problem in my life. I was on top of the BMX world and magazines labeled me "leader of the new school." I knew that I had some sort of established position in the industry. I'm not saying that I was the best in the world but I definitely built it up in my head that I had made it to a certain point. All these injuries, one after another, made me think, "You know what? You're killing yourself out here. You're in this position. You have support. Let's just kick back and do some other things while doing this." I spent a five year period where I rode my bike but didn't have the passion, didn't have the drive, to be doing it to its potential. All because I had these injuries stacking up and I thought, "I don't want to do another 360 tail whip because I know what that feels like if I mess up." Because of these injuries and not having the immune system I once had, I had to learn things that a doctor would have to know. I became so conscious of every little bit of food I put in my mouth and body and every little thing I do with myself. It allowed me to really, really understand the human body—book after book, article after article online, anything I could find. It drew my attention to what the human body can do on a daily basis that can make me the most efficient human I can be.

As of January 2009, I owned a vegan coffee shop, so I did my thing for a little while, maintained my BMX career, but not to its potential. All that came from this injury—from being hurt, trying not to be on pharmaceutical drugs all the time, having the injured spleen, and always getting sick.

Since then, I've re-entered my industry and I entered it with a positive mindset; a conscious, decision-making mindset where every move and every trick is well thought out. I have so much knowledge from what I unconsciously did for so long; it's all like muscle memory. Let's just say I'm doing a box jump. I've been jumping them for 18 years, and now I'm getting to a point where I'm trying to figure out the exact feeling it takes to maximize the amount of height, the amount of tricks, anything I can do on that one box jump instead of just jumping it for fun. I'm exploring new places like how relaxed I can be when I hit the ground with my two tires. I'm fully aware of all that. When something bad happens, something good always comes out of it. But it took so long. I'm 29 now and it took such a mindful way of thinking and I think it's because of my diet and because I'm doing things to better prepare myself.

I've been vegetarian for 13 years and vegan for 7. My reason for being vegetarian is different from my reason for being vegan. My vegetarianism is a compassionate thing. There is a level of compassion when it comes to milk, cheese, and eggs. But I found through diet and exercise and that I definitely don't want to consume any type of dairy products because I feel like it slows my body down. I have a laundry list of reasons it doesn't work for me.

I don't judge people if it works for them. My veganism is for me only. **I don't do it to make someone else do it. I do it for me**.

Eggs are something I chose to stop eating so I could be a full-blown vegan. Recently when I moved to California, I wanted to change things up. I did it in order to live in an environment where I am 100 percent in my option, where weather isn't a restriction, and my body is always at the same temperature. In yoga, you often hear that you move into a class by burning the inner flame within your core. That inner flame is very low in the winter because it's so cold in Chicago; your daily inner flame is not strong enough because you constantly have to prepare yourself, burn it, and then work out. When I'm in California, my body is at a warm temperature and is always somewhat ready to be worked out. I can go right into yoga and start stretching and not feel like I have a cramp or anything. There's no preparation in order to work out which I feel works so well for healing.

I was talking to Brian Kachinsky who is going through a knee surgery at the moment and I told him, "Look, I really think you need to be in a warm climate. Spend six months in California." He has his reasons for being here in Chicago. Obviously he lives here and wants to work it out but I feel like he has to spend 15 to 20 extra minutes getting to the point he needs to get to in order to actually work the leg out.

Along with moving to California, I feel like breathing is one of the most important parts of life. Obviously you can't live without it. I found myself in Chicago constantly doing neti pots, which is a salt water cleanse through your nasal system. One day I woke up thinking, "How can I eliminate this task? I need to be in an environment where allergies aren't giving me mental and physical stress every day." In California, I live right next to the ocean, breathing in salt water. That salt water makes me so clear; I can breathe now. I don't have to take any pharmaceutical drugs and I don't have to do neti pots every day. It keeps me on my toes and as energetic as I can be for that stretch of the day. Honestly, because I don't have any of those mental stresses, it's opening my mind to be able to ride, act, understand better, and be more aware. It's crazy and it's all from making a small adjustment in my life. **I feel like I can live off nothing because I'm so happy with what I've accomplished and who I am today.**

I've tried every different type of exercise. I found yoga is probably *the* best when it comes to my industry. People can argue with me about that. I feel like it's a balance. Your entire body needs to be balanced from head to toe, physically and mentally.

About nine years ago I started doing yoga and never really realized until the last two years how influential the teachings of yoga are in BMX, skateboarding, and anything in general. Earlier I talked about being conscious. That's the entire point of yoga: to be conscious of the present moment so you're aware of every move you make. Yoga is about finding the present balance in your mind and body.

I've been applying everything I've learned to my riding and I'm seeing remarkable similarities. It's working out to my advantage because I'm learning how to be more relaxed and to meditate on the thing that I'm about to do. One of the challenges BMX presents is that you're not physically capable of pulling off an actual trick because of its complications. It's so hard to understand why you can't get your pedal to slide across the rail. You've seen it done. A million people have done it but you can't do it. If you stop, breathe, think about it, take away the stresses that you may have for falling and you actually calculate it in your mind and meditate on the rail, you'll slide right across it. You just put your physical body to use using your brain's relaxation methods and you'll breeze right on the rail. You can bring that into any kind of position.

As far as healing, every day you go to yoga, you basically go through your body's entire network. From Downward Dog to Child's Pose to being upside down, stretching to the side, to the left, cobra poses—you feel every single inch of your body. If one leg is stronger than the other leg and if you go to yoga every single day, both legs will become equally as strong. If you have that balance, it's going to help with anything you do on your bike or skateboard. I'm right-handed so I tend to spin to the right. I'm spinning my head, shoulders, and body, and it's making me twist; a piece of metal is restricting me from twisting naturally, so I'm actually twisting my body so abruptly that I'm throwing my entire balance off. I'm building so much strength going right, but when I go left, it's a solid block. Since I started doing yoga every day about three months ago and *because* I do it every single day, I'm starting to see that when I do an opposite 360, which I used to be terrible at, I have the relaxation and strength to pull all the way around and it doesn't feel that off balance when I go right. And it's getting easier. The more I do this, the more I understand just how important it is to get off your bike and work out the muscles the bike doesn't work out.

Since I do yoga every day, my ankles, hips, calves, knees—everything is beginning to become perfectly in line. That's something I feel a lot of people in our industry need to know and understand. Again, this is just my opinion. What I'm doing is working for me and I hope people see that. I've had arguments with weight-lifting vert riders and they tell me that the heavier and stronger you are, the easier it is to adjust in the air. But then you see people like Tom Dugan, who's throwing down, breaking world records on a vert ramp, going high, and he's as pasty and as thin as you can be. He's lightweight and tall, but he's so flexible and relaxed when he rides that I can honestly see him busting a world record in half. If you put his honest effort together and he was completely relaxed, I could see him going 35 feet high or something. (Maybe that's ridiculous. I think the world record is 26, but he jumped the MegaRamp with ease at 18 feet and was just laughing about it the whole way up.) You know what Tom does? *Yoga.* He just chills. He's a really light, super happy guy. I feel like the riders and skaters in this world that accomplish the most are relaxed and easy-minded and so simple with their bodies, I can just see records being broken. Being able to completely control who you are and what you do—I think that's where you're going to find the real accomplishments.

I'm happy to say that I've been two years solid without any serious injury. I've been keeping a strong mental focus on my riding, trying to make sure that every single thing I do is consciously done. That's been my mission: to stay as healthy as possible.

In addition to staying focused and aware when it comes to riding or skating, you get so excited about the things you learn that you'll do 15 tricks in a row. You're not really intentionally doing it, but just kind of feeling and going with it. Today, my mentality is to treat each thing as its own, one trick at a time. I may move through them very quickly but I'm very aware of every movement I make.

There's been many times where I've created a new trick or done something different and people see it and they recognize me for it. But the enjoyment I get out of it is seeing a 15-year-old kid randomly doing it in front of me where he may have learned it from someone else. Knowing that I had something to do with that gives me the need to go on. **It's about bringing joy to other people and knowing I was there for the journey. That's who I am and that's what my riding is all about.**

I love to travel and the thought of traveling to a place where I can set a goal has always been glowing in my head. There's more to traveling than just the actual moving on foot to a different place. It's about your diet, injuries, moving somewhere, and trying to achieve a goal in your life. Maybe you smoke cigarettes, and want to quit smoking. What I tried doing my entire life is appreciate what I'm doing at the time because there's gonna be a time that I'm gonna reach the end of that. This is a quote that I've lived by my entire life: "Always draw a path for your journey but never anticipate the end of the journey because the journey itself is the goal." The goal is not at the end. It happens in between. That's something that I live by: appreciating every single moment that I'm in. It's called manifestation. As long as it's always there and always in your mind, it's something that will come into your life if you're moving in that direction.

Jerimiah just flat out rips! I've never seen Blunt Slides executed so fearlessly. About a year ago, Jerimiah and I did an interview where he poured his heart out to me. I was touched. I asked him not to touch me anymore. Beyond that though, he is seriously one of the nicest and talented guys in the world.

One of my best mini-ramp sessions to this day involved watching Jerimiah and Steve Fauser one evening. They were skating my ramp and killed it— so many tricks at blazing speeds. The ramp we called the Carwash was never the same after that. If inanimate objects have "spank banks," the biggest deposit was definitely made that night.

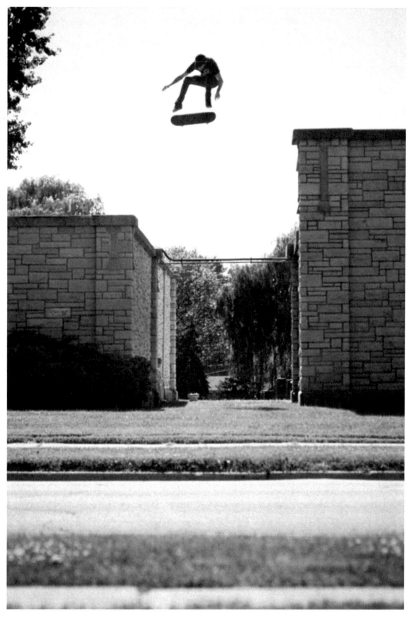

Jerimiah Smith   Photo: Ely Phillips

JERIMIAH SMITH

"A man is judged on the company he keeps, therefore, I'm screwed."

—Self Quote

26

SKATEBOARDER

17 YEARS SKATING

HOMETOWN: BOULDER CREEK, CA

CURRENT LOCATION: CHICAGO, IL

My name is Jerimiah Smith and I'm from a small town in the Santa Cruz Mountains in California called Bonny Doon. I got a skateboard for Christmas from my father when I was 11 years old. **I didn't have any cement where I lived so my dad laid down plywood for me to skate on just so I could have flat ground**. I never saw anyone skateboard at that point and I didn't really have any friends that were into it. Shortly after I got that first skateboard, my dad and I moved down the hill to a small town called Boulder Creek, with a population of only 2,500 people. It didn't have much cement either but I was still in heaven. Once I moved down there, I met another kid who skated by the name of

Micah Szoke. From then on out, the rest is history. I couldn't put it down and I really can't say that I will ever be able to.

Skateboarding has taken a pretty heavy toll on my body. I've had a lot of back issues as of late. I wouldn't change a thing that I did but at the same time it's wearing me down mentally as well. I think about it every day. I'd like to do something about it but I'm a pretty stubborn bastard and I'll probably live with the pain for the rest of my life.

 I've broken my nose, tailbone, wrist, ankle, been knocked out multiple times, had multiple sprains and strains keeping me off my board for months, torn my meniscus and had knee surgery, just to name a few.

The one injury that stands out in my mind the most was when I tore the lateral meniscus in my knee. Now, it wasn't the most painful of injuries or even the longest recovery time. It was something about the fact that I had to have surgery, spend a shit ton of money, have something removed from my body, do physical therapy, and rely on my friends to take care of me. I'm sure things could have been a lot worse but I'm not used to people taking care of me or having to take care of myself for that matter. **Physical therapy was a good "training" process for me, teaching myself to take care of my body and actually getting myself back to "normal."** Since this injury was a little more serious than ones in the past, it put a new light in my eyes and taught me that if you take good care of your body it will treat you right in the end. Imagine that, right?

If you skateboard, there isn't one thing you can do to prevent an injury; it's just a fact. That's how you know when people skate seriously and have done it for many years: they must love it with a passion. I've never had a routine to healing other than hating my life while I can't skate and drinking as many beers as I can to make the mental pain go away.

What a story! When Mary and I first talked I was blown away. You've got *huh*? You're how old? You're doing what? I was full of questions and knew right away that she would be gracing the pages here. Mary is a warrior and survivor. She is 98 percent black woman and two percent machine; she is a virtual soul cyborg! When you look at the photo, take a look at the left knee.

She is the future. *Plus*, her kids will always be able to say,

"My Mom surfs better than your mom!"

Enough said.

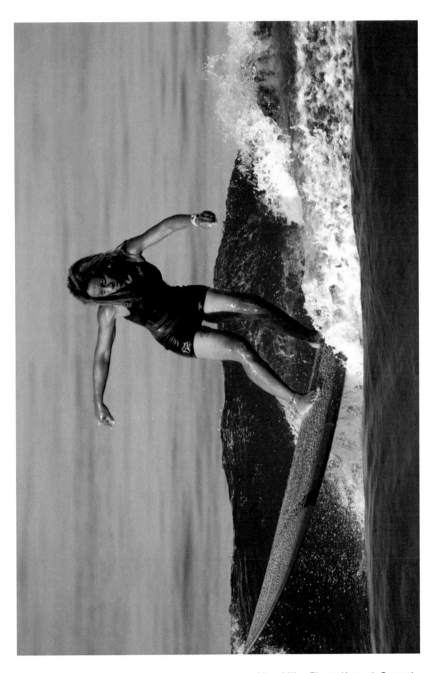

Mary Mills   Photo: Kenneth Samuels

MARY MILLS

"Just do it." —Nike

48

SURFER

9 YEARS SURFING

HOMETOWN: LOS ANGELES, CA

CURRENT LOCATION: LOS ANGELES, CA

Little black girls didn't surf when I was a kid. In fact, little black girls with straightened hair didn't go near water. *Ever.* It was, and still is for many, all about the hair. But I don't give a damn about hair. At 12, I fell in love with surfing and skateboarding . . . even though I couldn't swim and didn't do the former, and was forbidden by my parents to do the latter. I used to sneak away to skate, and I'd always get caught. *Always.* As if that wasn't bad enough, I spent much of my adolescence being questioned by my peers about my choices. Black girls didn't wear Vans and ride skateboards. That's what white people did. That's what white *boys* did. Nevertheless, I continued to love both pursuits for decades even when I wasn't pursuing them.

Then, at 39, I had a child. By that point, I had cut off all my hair and learned to swim. I was a fish that still wanted to surf. When my son was about three or four months old, I began learning how to surf and have been surfing seriously ever since. It was also around that time that an orthopedist told me a knee replacement was in my future. I hadn't realized that it would be the near future.

In 2009, when I was 45, my knee was done. A massive soccer injury at 17 had led to me to this place. Although I feared the outcome, I had the surgery within a month of being told I needed it. Three and a half months later, I was back on my surfboards.

I assumed my health would be considered excellent given my age and my status as someone with a titanium joint. I do everything I want to do within reason. I recognize that my joint is one which doctors think I should be a bit careful. With that said, I seem to slam at the skate park quite a bit. The knee can take it.

I think the fact that I'm mindful of my age and that I have to work hard (by lifting weights and eating right) to play hard (i.e., surfing and skating and whatever else I do) helps in the long run. I know I'm not a kid anymore, but I swear I'm having much more fun than I did 20 years ago. I think I'm equally as fit too. I may have lost a step here and there, but I have not lost much muscle, drive, or stoke.

At 17, while playing soccer in college, I suffered a massive injury to my left knee. It was so bad that I heard everything tear, as did the two women who hit me. I eventually had two operations to repair the damage and just went on with my athletic life. I couldn't play soccer after that, but I did end up doing things like racing bikes and running marathons.

That knee was never quite right. Still, I always worked with it and around it. I'm a big believer in just dealing with the hand you're dealt. **Life's too short to lament things you can't change.** I couldn't turn back the clock and prevent that knee injury from occurring. So, I lived with it. However, the knee got progressively more painful over the years. It got to the point where I didn't want to surf. That's when I knew something was very, very wrong.

I went to an orthopedist, hoping he wouldn't say it was time for a knee replacement while knowing in my heart of hearts that he would. And he did. I was stunned, certain my life as a surfer was over. I went home and cried. Then I decided to get it done. I was already in too much pain to surf. That pain was only going to get worse. I realized the knee replacement was my only hope.

Recovering from a knee replacement is painful as fuck! It truly is! Initially, the pain was more intense than anyone could have told me. It's like some horrible form of torture—having the ends of your bones cut off and capped with titanium. The pain slowly decreased, but it seemed like the knee just didn't want to work.

There was a great deal of doubt and angst in my recovery because I just could not fathom this skinny, scarred, and horribly painful joint ever being up to the task of surfing again. I think it's worse for someone who's active. Most people with knee replacements just want to be rid of the pain. Now that the surgery is being done on those of us who are younger and younger, you're finding that many of us need it in order to return to our lives.

I think what helped me is that I tend to be on the stubborn side when it comes to doing the things I love and I also have a high threshold for pain. I went off the prescription pain meds by the second or third week; they seemed to do more damage than good. Then, I gave up on the over-the-counter meds because of their potential damage to my organs. What really helped me get through the pain was medical marijuana and ice. I used the former to help me sleep. And if you can get some sleep through the recovery process, you're golden.

I just set a goal for when I wanted to be back on the surfboard. It wasn't a hard and fast one, but it was something I could shoot for. I think I got back on the board a week after my target day. It wasn't easy; it was just a matter of knowing I could do it.

I've learned that I'm a badass! I guess I kind of knew it, but the knee replacement solidified that understanding. I had a knee replacement and then started surfing three and a half months later! And this is with no real role models with regard to surfing and knee replacement. I found one surfer on the Internet who had a knee replacement, but I didn't have a lot of details about what he went through. That's why I was diligent about including my experiences in my surf blog. I wanted to leave a paper (or I guess, electronic) trail for those who would follow behind me. I wanted others to know that they could return to surfing after the surgery.

I am much more appreciative of my health since the knee replacement. You'd never know this by how much I fall down at the skate park! **I feel like the knee has given me a new lease on life. Without it, I would no longer be an athlete; I'd be disabled, fat, in pain, and in a bad way.** But doctors can rebuild us! For that, I am grateful to live at this time in history.

As for preventing injuries, I guess that depends on your attitude. When I skate, I don't push it the way I might have prior to the knee replacement and prior to middle age. I try to do enough so that if I fall, I won't seriously break anything. I lift weights like a fiend. I recognize that muscle protects joints. As someone who surfs and skates, I know I'm putting my joints through some serious stress. I figure muscle is the best way to protect them from the stress that I put on them (whether it be paddling hard for hours or falling hard off the skateboard).

I've pretty much stopped eating meat. I think that's made me healthier. I eat it maybe once a month. I feel a lot lighter now that I don't eat meat.

I do stretch quite a bit now. Skating has made me realize how necessary this is. I've paid attention to my surfing muscles for so long that skating made me see how much I'd neglected my lower body (even though I raced bikes for many years). It's easy to pull muscles when you skate; therefore, I do some serious stretching for my lower body now.

I don't want to write Timmy's intro (sigh). This cat is one of my best friends and this has bias written all over it. We skate together several times a week, play in the same band, have the same girlfriend...I mean, his girlfriend is a good friend, you know. We talk, laugh, break bread, and philosophize together on a *regular* basis.

Besides being a good friend and a damn good person or human, as he would say, he is also an awesome skateboarder. In it for all the right reasons, karma is not a bitch, but an angel. Even before the age of 20, one of his main priorities was reaching out to younger kids through skateboarding, rapping, and breakdancing.

Selflessness is a rare quality. Not only does it reward Timmy's being but also feeds those around him with inspiration as well.

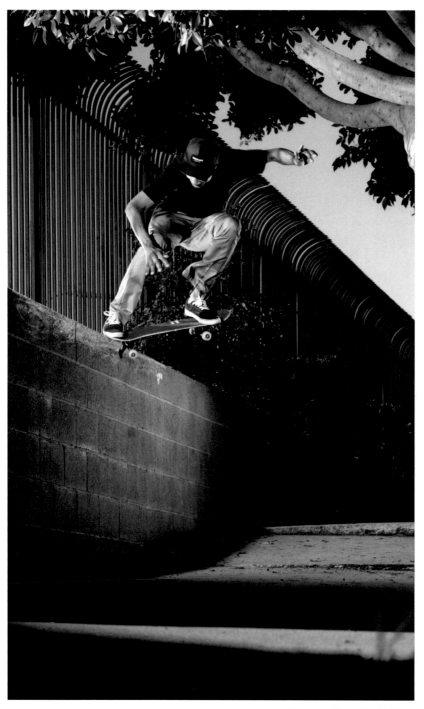

Timothy Johnson   Photo: Ely Phillips

TIMMY JOHNSON

"To be loved is as important as a mother's touch is to her child."

—Self Quote

21

AM SKATEBOARDER

13 YEARS SKATEBOARDING

HOMETOWN: CHICAGO, IL

CURRENT LOCATION: CHICAGO, IL

I'm a member of the most innovative, inspirational, progressive, most watched, most hated, and most loved skateboard online video series called *T.C. Mixtapes*.

As of now, I feel like I'm in good physical health. I'm not that active in terms of skateboarding (due to the weather) but I stay moving and workout often. Mentally, I'm prepared to jump down twenty stairs and skate all day, every day, but I do feel out of tune and would need to put in some hard practice hours to feel 100 percent on my board. I would say mentally I'm there 100 percent and physically I'm there only 75. Also, I sprained my ankle on October 5 [2011] and it still hurts as I type.

One time I tried a laser heel flip off this launch ramp that sent me about 15 feet high and I landed on my feet on concrete. I tried the trick for four hours. **On one of the attempts, I was about to land the board but it didn't flip all the way and I landed primo which gave me the biggest bruise on the bottom of my left foot, keeping me off the board for a month.** I couldn't walk for a couple of days.

Another time, I was skating downtown with the Uprise Crew. We skated for about three or so hours cruising the streets, hitting up different spots, and at the end of the session, I sat down for about twenty minutes. When I stood up to say goodbye to peeps and go home, my knee got really inflamed. I didn't tweak, hit, or bang my knee; it just blew up and it was hard for me to walk. That took me out the game for a month or so.

I didn't really do much for either of my injuries. With my knee I just didn't skate and tried to massage the fluid out. There was no change in my diet. I usually eat healthy but I didn't try to eat certain things to aid in the process. I went to the doctor and got X-rays but never got the results. The doctor told me that it was probably an inflamed tendon and I would be okay.

It was the same thing with my foot bruise. I iced and elevated it to help the swelling go down. My method of healing was to not skate.

I live a stress-free life and I think that helped in my healing process. I do feel like these injuries have made me stronger.

I think stretching is important because it loosens up the muscles and gives you more rebound. Let's say you didn't stretch and your breaking point is 45 degrees. You are more likely to break something than an individual who did stretch and has a breaking point of 90 degrees. Some people can even stretch beyond that to about 200 degrees. Being a skateboarder and having a high rebound is important because we're constantly hitting the ground, bending, pushing, etc.

To prevent injury, I think practice is important as well as being realistic about what you're capable of doing. It's almost like watching a movie of one guy beating up 50 guys. In your head you might say to yourself, "If I was in that situation I would win," but realistically, 50-to-1 is a no-brainer. Same goes with trying a skateboard trick. You may look at video of pros flying down 20 stairs and rails and feel like you can do the same and you *can* (there's nothing wrong with confidence), but you must take little steps. Skate the five stair first and work your way up. Personally, I still enjoy it and feel it is important to skate flat ground or train on a five stair because it gives me more control and helps me become consistent; once that happens, I take it to the big stairs.

When it comes to healing from an injury, just try to relax and stay productive mentally. Try not to stress if you can't do what you were doing before. Use that time to work on other things and get prepared for a new day.

I do think eating properly while injured is important because in the event you sprain your ankle, for example, your body automatically sends extra help to that part of your body to care of it. On top of spraining your ankle, let's say you eat a big fried chicken dinner with potatoes and a big slice of cake for dessert. Along with your body trying to care for your ankle, now your body is working even harder to digest the food at the same time. I think eating foods like fruits and veggies is important because those foods also send help to places in need and doesn't take too much time for your body to digest.

I try to have a balanced diet and eat fruits and veggies as much as I can, but I still eat junk food. When I'm out skating and I don't stretch, all I think about is getting hurt. But when I take the time to stretch, I feel more confident in my abilities. Off and on I take glucosamine, fish oil, and flax seed oil (thanks Soma). I try to listen to relaxing music that relieves stress. I also break dance. Breakdancing helps with my skateboarding because it gets me used to being on the ground. So if I ever happen to fall, which doesn't usually happen, I can use those breakdance skills to maneuver properly on the ground.

If you look on the next page you'll see why Ray spends every day on the slopes practicing. Oh wait. No, it's a *courthouse* where Ray spends all his time. Hmmmm, I forgot about that! Ray Lang is hereby officially deemed "one of the busiest fuckers I know." This guy puts in work. For someone to have been through what he's been through, you would well expect him to be some rich fat fart sitting around with an ugly tie and a fine wife. Instead, he can't be stopped, has some sense of fashion, and actually does have a fine wife. Yeah I know, my second time referring to someone's significant other. Won't happen again!

Like all the others in this chapter, he is a winner, point blank. Ray kicks ass on snow or concrete. By the way, that photo and knowing the man in it is one of the many inspirations for *Tough Like You*. I'll let Ray take it from here.

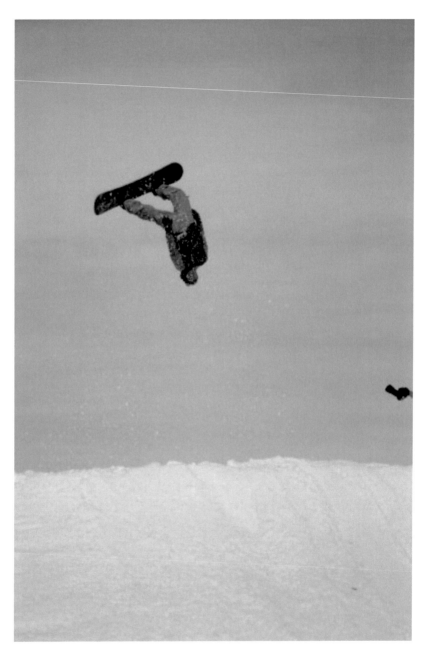

Ray Lang   Photo: Travis Feiss

RAY LANG

"If I ever start to get sour about how much pain I'm in, or that I'm skating seven stair handrails instead of 14, I just think of Cardiel and what he's been through, and it gives me some perspective really quickly." —Self Quote

36

SNOWBOARDER/SKATEBOARDER

25 YEARS BOARDING

HOMETOWN: ST. LOUIS, MO

CURRENT LOCATION: CHICAGO, IL

I was born in 1975 in St. Louis, Missouri. As a child, I always gravitated toward activities with a daredevil element. When I was four years old, I wanted to be Evil Knievel when I grew up. After spending the first part of my childhood trying to see how far I could jump my BMX bike, I got my first skateboard at age 11. Much like Chicago, St. Louis is not very conducive to skateboarding in the winter, so in 1987 I figured that snowboarding would be the next best thing. That very first winter I found that not only did snowboarding give me something to do in the winter, but I loved being out there just as much as I loved skateboarding. Like most dual skateboarder/snowboarders, snowboarding allowed me to do all of the things I wish I could do on a skateboard. As a result of being so much easier than skateboarding, the scale of speed, jumps, tricks, and rails were significantly larger, and as a result, more dangerous.

After snowboarding for four years, I got sponsored by my local shop. In 1994 during my senior year in high school, my shop got me sponsored by a couple different companies. After high school I went right into college; however, I scheduled my classes so that I could travel as much as I could all winter. I'd drive myself out West for large blocks of time, couch surfing wherever I was welcome.

In February 1998, I was in a snowboarding contest. During that contest, I overshot a jump and ruptured the discs in my lower back. That was the last day I was ever able to do anything at 100 percent. In 2003, I graduated from law school. I've been practicing law as a trial lawyer for the past eight years.

The most significant injury I've had is the ruptured discs in my lower back. Every day, no matter what I'm doing, I experience pain and discomfort in my lower back. I've lost a good deal of flexibility and cold weather locks me up almost completely. Sitting at a desk for most of my day doesn't help. I have to get up five or six times a day, close my office door, and lay on the floor so my back can unwind. Whether it's skateboarding, snowboarding, or any physical activity, I cannot function at the level or in the way I want.

It's been almost 14 years since the fall that blew out my back and for the most part I've just learned to live with it, but it takes a mental toll on me as well. It's frustrating not being able to skateboard and snowboard at the level I know I would have been able. Despite my physical condition, I stay pretty positive. I remain thankful that at 36 years old I'm still able to participate in the sports that I love and that my injuries aren't more serious or debilitating.

My major injuries include the following: three ruptured discs in my back, between levels L3–S1; a broken right ulna; separated right shoulder; completely torn left shoulder; broken and dislocated thumb; around ten concussions, three of those being pretty serious; significant arthritis in my lower back, both feet, and both shoulders; and some strange medical phenomenon where my right elbow is always swollen.

Rupturing the discs in my back was a major turning point in my life. Within the five minutes following that crash, I couldn't move a muscle without lightning bolts of pain shooting through my entire body. I couldn't get myself out of bed, or even a chair, without having something to help pull myself up. **When I felt a sneeze coming on I'd grab something to squeeze and prepared for hell.** After a couple weeks of not being able to put on my own socks and shoes, I finally got my first in a series of cortisone epidurals. The cortisone was a godsend. After the first shot I could function pretty well. After all three epidurals I felt well enough to begin rehabilitation, which consisted of strengthening my core and lifting weights for the first time in my life. I also began paying attention to my diet and nutrition.

Several months after I started lifting weights, I felt pretty good. Not only was my back pain significantly reduced, but I was getting a lot stronger all over. In fact, by the time the next winter came around I thought I was back to 100 percent. Shortly into that winter, however, I learned that the structure of my spinal cord had been compromised, and the heavy demand and impacts I had subjected myself to were no longer possible. The next three years were a constant cycle of injury and rehabilitation, until in 2001 when I couldn't skate or snowboard at all. I was forced to take more than five years away from snowboarding completely, focusing solely on weight training and rehabilitation.

In 2007, I slowly got back into snowboarding. Little by little I worked my way back up to where I was having fun again. With regular cardio and taking up yoga, in 2009 I was able to skateboard again for the first time in nine years.

Blowing out my lower back changed the course of my life, no question about it. In fact, it prevented me from accomplishing a great number of dreams and goals I'd set for myself. But I never regretted it even for a second. It's just the nature of the beast. Being involved in skateboarding at a high level, and especially snowboarding, is accompanied by great risk. If top level snowboarding wasn't dangerous, everyone would be a pro. My willingness to take risks ultimately resulted in blowing out my back, but it also got me to where I was on that day. You've got to take the good with the bad, and in my particular case, this was the hand I was dealt. In my experience with just about everything in life, you regret those things you don't do far more than the things you do (in fact, that's probably a bumper sticker). While I'll deal with physical pain for the rest of my life, I have peace of mind knowing that I gave it my all; that's a fair trade to me. A lot of people don't understand that, and that's okay.

John Cardiel got injured five years after me, but he is still a huge inspiration. Cards was better at both sports than I ever would have been anyway, and today he's not able to participate in either, at all. Regardless, he's as positive as can be and chooses to find what's still good in his life. If I ever start to get sour about how much pain I'm in, or that I'm skating seven stair handrails instead of 14, I just think of Cardiel and what he's been through, and it gives me some perspective really quickly. **Live every day to the fullest and be thankful for what you have.** All hail Cardiel!

Carefully monitoring my weight and what I eat seems to be more important every year I get older. Even if I gain five pounds, it makes a big difference in the pain I feel and in how well I'm able to move around. I stay away from processed foods and limit my carbohydrate intake. Most of what I eat is natural food, never frozen or preserved. My diet is high in protein, and usually covered in hot sauce.

I supplement my diet with a good amount of fish oil, calcium, and a multivitamin. The fish oil seems to help my joints a great deal. Before my injury, I never bothered to stretch at all. Now I am forced to stretch religiously or I tighten up quickly. I have a 30-minute yoga DVD that I practice in the laughter-free environment of my home, and it seems to keep me out there.

Matt Frankland is not the Matt Frankland as labeled in his e-mail address. Here's another person much too close to me to *not* write subjectively. He is a very dear friend. If I didn't know him that well, I might say something like, "damn that dude's got some crazy ass Hard Flips" or maybe I would just criticize and hate on his old beat-up truck.

Like Timmy, this is the person I've skated with the most in the last few years. We meet up downtown or at a park and just rip for hours, talk about life, and rip some more. Even though I only know .01 percent of the tricks he does, we somehow manage to have the most intense sessions that usually end with us both feeling my age. Matt skates hard and doesn't know the meaning of a mellow session. If he can't roll fast and intense, he'll opt to just sit and chill. The man has a need for speed. He also has a need for numbers. With a master's degree in economics, he lives the duality of corporate life and skater rat.

The only person to have a key to my building (because I grew weary frequently throwing mine out the window), I look forward to many more years rippin' with Matt.

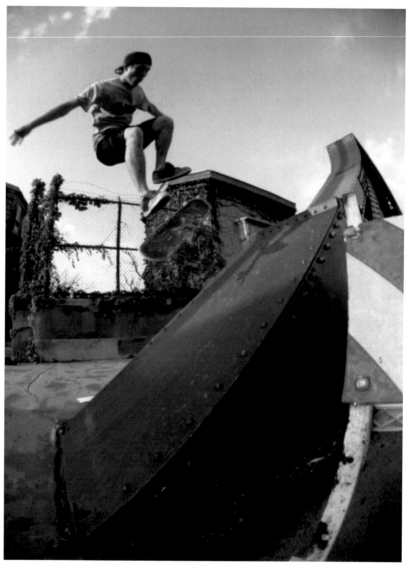

Matt Frankland   Photo: Charles Crawford

MATT FRANKLAND

"Try to land your trick every time. Go fast & don't complain."
—Self Quote

25

SKATEBOARDER

13 YEARS SKATEBOARDING

HOMETOWN: RIVER GROVE, IL

CURRENT LOCATION: CHICAGO, IL

I was born on my parents' living room floor in 1986. I've been skateboarding since I was 12 and riding road bikes since I was 19. I'm not going pro anytime soon and that's fine because I skate for the love of it, and Chicago takes care of me. I've spent over half of my life obsessing over that useless wooden plank and the feeling of stepping on it and pushing forward gets me every time. I have to warn girls when I start dating them to not interfere with my skateboarding because, "I've known my skateboard far longer than you, and my skateboard never does me wrong."

My road bike, on the other hand, is happy playing second fiddle to my skateboard. I started biking after I moved to Chicago for college. I did it first as a way to get around, but now it is one of my favorite things to do. I changed my daily commute from the worst part of my day to the best—rain or shine, snow or wind, it doesn't matter.

I'm very healthy right now. Luckily I have a job where I can sit at a desk all day and recover.

I've been lucky enough to know my limits and I've never broken a bone (knock on wood). However, I was a slouch throughout school, and as a kid I always thought my body was resilient enough to handle anything I wanted. Sometime around 22 years old, I paid the price.

It was a warm, late November day in Chicago. It was also finals week for me, and I was skating hard outside every day, no warm-ups, trying to soak in the last of the skate year before winter set and we were stuck with the indoor parks until March.

Well there was no one trick that did it; my lower back slowly gave up on me. **I remember trying so hard to ignore the pain and keep on skating, but I couldn't even crouch down to do tricks**. My back was throbbing with pain and I began walking stiff as a board.

At the time, I worked at a retail store on the sales floor, and my back would throb so bad that I would have to hide the pain from customers by walking away for a second just to lean on a wall and rest. The pain became so powerful that it shot down my legs and my entire lower half would go back and forth between numbness and excruciating pain. I couldn't stand up for more than five minutes without collapsing and I feared it would be the end of my skate career. I refused to take pain pills or see a doctor for the entire month of December. I think I only went out partying once that month because of the pain.

I finally gave in and saw a doctor. He told me I had a slipped disc in my lower back, scoliosis in two different parts of my spine, and the herniated disc was pinching my sciatic nerve. The sciatic nerve runs from the top of your neck to your toes and it's the nerve highway for your entire body. That explained the throbbing pain in my legs.

The doctor gave me a couple cortisone shots and set me up with a physical therapist. I did three months of back exercises with old people at the local gym and I was all right. Although my back still acts up after a tough day of skating, I am very thankful to have had the experience I did. **Now I have a half hour stretch routine to get myself ready to skate, and I am much more in tune with how my body works.** I skate longer, I feel better afterward, and I know that I can skate for years to come.

I believe in having a sound body, mind, and soul. I love skateboarding to death—it's my religion and I'm a fanatic. The best thing you can do for any sport is stretch before and after. It doesn't matter how silly you look, you'll skate better, I promise.

I don't eat anything special. I have horrible eating habits because I've been blessed with a high metabolism. The only advice I can give is to eat a whole frozen pizza before you go skate because it gives you energy. I told you I had horrible eating habits.

One thing that really helped my skating was the transition to road biking as my primary mode of transportation. I get my daily exercise by riding my bike downtown to work every day (as opposed to the train/bus/car). One of the best things you can do with your day is ride a bike to work or school. It's free, faster (in Chicago at least), and turns all the boring, downtime of commuting into exercise.

I was on the side of 200 foot rock in Arizona when I yelled out to Stoyan Angelov that I was in trouble. As fit as I thought I was, my legs were freaking out. They were wobbling more and more uncontrollably and it was affecting my grasp on the rock. I was in a state of severe panic. I was a beginner at climbing to say the least and the term "sewing machine legs" was not yet in my vocabulary.

After what seemed like a lifetime but was actually only few seconds, Stoyan calmly said, "Take a break." I thought, "What the hell does 'take a break on a rock I'm about to fall off' mean, 'cookies and milk' time?" But like all good teachers, he was able to guide me to a much calmer state. That's right; it took Stoyan, who was several feet away, to remind me I was attached to specialized gear designed for me not to become coyote food. He coaxed me into planting my feet firmly on the rock, and to totally take my arms away from the rock and rope. I was extended almost straight out from the side.

At that moment looking down knowing that if something snapped, I was dead, I felt both scared and free at the same time. It was a new physical, mental, and emotional something that will never be forgotten.

To Stoyan, it was an easy climb strictly for teaching me the basics—that and a damn good way to give his father-in-law a fear-induced heart attack. I must have mumbled something about the insurance policy not being paid up before he helped me. An exceptional athlete in many disciplines, Stoyan is a beast.

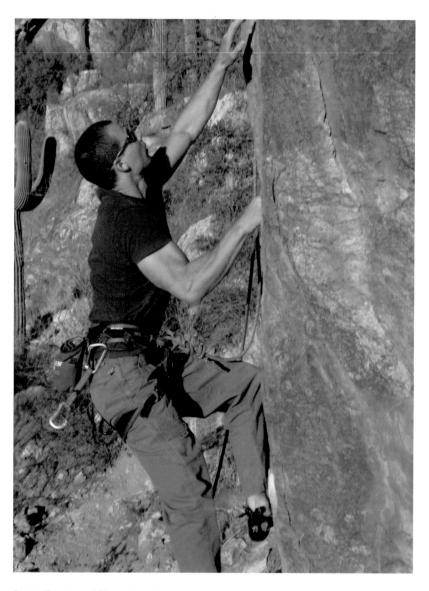

Photo: Courtesy of Stoyan Angelov

STOYAN ANGELOV

"He who suffers, remembers." —Unknown

29

ROCK/ICE/ALPINE CLIMBING AND TRIATHLON

12 YEARS CLIMBING & 7 TRIATHLON

HOMETOWN: SOFIA, BULGARIA

CURRENT LOCATION: TUCSON, ARIZONA

If there is one thing I can say for sure about myself, it is that I love the outdoors. I was practically born there. I was only six months old when my parents took me on my first camping trip. We weren't car camping either. I obviously don't remember the event but from what I was told, the trek to our first camp involved a shortcut through a train tunnel high in the mountains. Apparently the timing wasn't great, since somewhere in the middle of the tunnel we all had to hug the damp stone walls as the train cars whipped by only mere inches away. Anyway, you get the picture of what my childhood was like. While most kids watched *Looney Toons*, a few friends and I were out in the woods with a rope, pocket knife, and a set of matches (frequently without adult supervision). I learned to tie a figure eight knot before I learned which numbers added up to eight. Luckily, my parents always supported and encouraged my exploratory behavior, even when it was risky.

When I was 14, my family moved to Chicago and we spent a couple of years stuck in the city, learning the language and getting to know American culture. During my second year of high school, I was introduced to climbing and it completely took over my life. I spent the first year learning the ropes from a group of experienced friends and subsequently, over the next several years, took lengthy trips to many of the mountain states and overseas. It is tough for outsiders of the sport to appreciate the difficulties associated with climbing a technical peak or high wall.

First, there is the matter of being fit enough to get yourself and your gear to the base. Then there is the need for having the strength, endurance, and skill to complete the climb. Lastly, you still have to get down despite being frequently plagued by bad weather, darkness, fatigue, and gear management issues. The biggest part of the game, however, is in your head. **There is a complex mix of emotions associated with being in the middle of nowhere with no one but your partner to rely on.** I often experienced excitement, anxiety, fear, and happiness almost simultaneously. Buried deep in those experiences are valuable lessons to be learned and huge rewards in confidence and self-knowledge to be gained. I was beyond hooked. Fortunately, I survived the steep learning curve associated with being new to traditional outdoor climbing.

Another thing I have always liked is biology. Because of my love for climbing, I was able to align these two interests by learning about training and exercise physiology. After completing my undergraduate training in biology, I earned certification from the American College of Sports Medicine as a health fitness instructor. I worked in that capacity at Northeastern Illinois University as well as Northwestern University. Because my job as a trainer limited my time spent abroad, I had to adopt a rigorous and comprehensive training plan to maximize the transferability of my fitness during my climbing trips. It was during that time that I was introduced to my other passion: triathlons.

Endurance training is an integral part of climbing mountains. Somewhere in the long hours spent on a bike and running trails, I realized that there is much to be gained from diving into this new realm of sports that I previously considered much too urban for my liking. What followed were several years of an equally intense pursuit of both climbing endeavors and triathlon races. I started out with shorter races but quickly became obsessed with distance. My favorite race type became the half-distance Ironman Triathlon (1.2 mile swim, 56 mile bike, and 13.1 mile run). Ultimately, I built up to the full-distance Ironman Triathlon.

Here, I hit a turning point. The volume of training required to compete in Ironman triathlons left all other aspects of my fitness underdeveloped. I lost strength and muscle mass that was critical for the types of climbing I enjoyed most. At this time I also moved to Tucson, Arizona to begin my doctoral training in cardiovascular physiology, married my college sweetheart, and acquired a home. The intensity of academic work and new commitments in life left me with even less time to train and travel. During the first year, I struggled to find balance between my training and the rest of my life but thanks to support from my wife and friends, I found a great way to balance things out.

Though I rarely compete these days, my training and outdoor projects are every bit intense and rewarding. Arizona, as it turns out, is a very wild place. The mountains here offer no half days. There are thousands of remote, committing, highly technical, and mentally demanding climbs. As I write this in the winter of 2011, my climbing partner and I are training for a spring ascent of 1,000 foot route on a giant granite dome in the Santa Catalina Mountains. But the one thing that really brings me joy is that my wife and I have found a new way to utilize the little free time we have—we use our fitness, training, and climbing skills to give back to the outdoor community. **About 18 months ago, I joined the search and rescue team and after completing the nearly year-long training, I now participate (whenever I can) in rescuing people stranded or injured in the mountains**.

My physical health is excellent at the moment. I recovered from an injury suffered over a year ago in a trail accident (partially torn deltoid ligament). The initial injury came from shorting a jump while boulder-hopping out of a riverbed near camp, but what worsened the condition was the forced march out of the field with a heavy pack. The weather that day deteriorated and our group was forced to leave sooner (and move faster) then I wanted us to. Imaging did not reveal any fractures. I wore a plastic boot for about two weeks but eventually, this change in gait caused overuse and inflammation to the knee joint of the opposite leg. I began using crutches and subsequently recovered. The entire ordeal lasted several weeks.

My mental health is also quite good. I'm always coping with stress associated with juggling a very demanding career, home ownership, and rigorous training for action sports. Work can get quite overwhelming at times but my training and outdoor activities allow me to keep an even keel. The one thing I enjoy about climbing is that once the light goes green on a trip, the volume on everything else in my life gets turned down. It's hard to worry about work when you know you have more immediate problems (like not falling on a questionable piece of protection). Because safety in the mountains depends largely on preparation, the trip really starts in my living room where the gear is packed, checked, and rechecked. I visualize the entire plan, play the "what if" game, and only then finalize the selection. The whole experience from packing the gear to returning home requires intense concentration, which allows for an effective break from work. The whole process, from start to finish, is really quite meditative.

Overuse injuries:

Overuse injuries to the hands and arms are extremely common in climbers and in my early years, I was certainly no exception. During my first year, I climbed five to six days per week. I climbed indoor walls during the week and on the weekends I climbed outdoors as often as possible. It wasn't long before the volume and intensity started catching up with me. The first injury I suffered was inflammation to the proximal interphalangeal (PIP) joints. My fingers swelled and the pain, though dull and not particularly intense, frequently kept me up all night. Within weeks I got tendonitis of the forearm tendons as well. I tried taking two weeks off from climbing but within few days of starting back up, my symptoms returned. I ended up not climbing for two months and was only able to return very slowly (only climbing once or twice a week at first). The tendonitis did come back two more times after the subsequent year but I was able to fend off the symptoms by backing off from training at the first sign of trouble. Eventually, I found that my ideal climbing frequency is about three times per week. Consistent climbing and better climbing session frequency have allowed me to stay out of trouble with both conditions ever since.

In addition to the tendonitis and joint inflammation, I frequently struggled with flexibility and muscle strength imbalances. As a kid I was always a thinner, slow twitch muscle fiber, ectomorph kind of a guy. Flexibility was never my strong suit either. However, climbing allowed the muscles associated with pulling to over-develop in relation to the rest of my musculature. Consequently, I suffered frequent injuries to the shoulders and spasms in the lower back. After a while, I realized the benefits of a comprehensive strength training program aimed at improving performance of all muscles (climbing related and not). Strength training has been at the core of all my training since then.

Another notable overuse injury was caused by running a full marathon on two weeks notice. A friend of mine had signed up for a race but couldn't compete because of a family emergency. He asked if I would enjoy the event if he transferred the registration to me. Foolishly, I said yes. I had been cycling hard in 100 mile century rides that season and felt that there would be a great transferability of cardiovascular fitness. I was right, but not entirely. **While my muscular and cardiovascular endurance were more than adequate, my tendons and ligaments were not adapted to the higher impact associated with running (as opposed to cycling). I was plagued by knee pain for the next year and a half**. Eventually, a consistent running schedule solved the problem. I never ran long distances again without gradually building up first.

Accident-associated injuries:

A laundry list of my accident injuries reads as follows: one concussion, a soft tissue injury of the lateral deltoid, soft tissue injury to the right forearm, sprain of the right shoulder, more ankle sprains then I care to count, and one very notable occasion when I drove the front point of my ice climbing crampon into my calf muscle. Most of these were suffered in bike crashes and climbing falls. Luckily, I've never broken a single bone. Probably the worst accident I ever had was in the summer of 2004. I was struck by an SUV while cycling. Due to the heat and humidity that day, I had opted out of wearing either a shirt or a helmet. My bike was sucked under the SUV and I went airborne over the handlebar.

After practically being mummified by the ambulance crew, I spent five very uncomfortable hours at the ER. On the list of possible injuries were: a cracked skull, cracked vertebral column, broken ribs, broken arm, muscle tears, and many others. We all watched with relief and amusement as the X-rays and MRIs came back clean. Amazingly, I was out with just a concussion, a few moderate muscle injuries to the upper body, and lots of road rash. The doctor credited the lack of more serious injuries to a good roll, dense bones, low body weight, and a hardcore group of guardian angels. One benefit of this accident is that I never go on a training ride without a helmet anymore—that thing is glued to my skull.

If you are an action athlete, you are going to get hurt at some point. Period. It's just a cold, hard game of statistics. Each attempt to pull off a hard rock climb, skate trick, or sick mountain bike line carries high probability of failure. By the very nature of the sport you will fail more times than you succeed. If you are a climber and you never fall, then you are not climbing hard enough. If you are never nervous before a trip then your projects aren't challenging enough. Thus, injuries due to accidents and mishaps are inevitable in action sports.

So now that you know with mathematical certainty you are going to get hurt, how do you prepare? How do you stack the odds in order to ensure minimal damage when you do take a bad fall, get stuck on a peak in bad weather, or get your leg broken in a rock fall? Wearing protective gear is a good start, as is honing your aerial skills (think tuck and roll), meticulous equipment maintenance, and careful planning. However, I firmly believe that in any sport, fitness is the true basis for safety. Having a robust musculoskeletal system and good cardiovascular fitness will go a long way to prevent injuries and speed recovery.

Remember all of those muscle imbalance issues I mentioned earlier? For me, they were profound. Let me elaborate. Early in my climbing, the biggest sources of injury stemmed from weak (and inflexible) lower back, chest, and anterior deltoid muscles. I suffered from frequent shoulder pain and spasms in my lower back. These kept coming back no matter how I adjusted the frequency, intensity, or duration of my climbing. To be completely honest, I first started strength training because I thought it would make me a better climber. Initially, I trained the pulling muscles but later adopted a much more comprehensive program. As I experimented with different programs, I eventually found out what worked and what didn't. Truth be told, there is so much information out there that it can get overwhelming. There are virtually endless questions. How many sets? How many reps? What is the ideal frequency? Should I use split routines or not? What periodization scheme should I use? It goes on and on. It took me years to sort it all out.

When I did, though, the results were amazing. Once I was able to fit all my training into a systematic year-round periodization program, I never suffered from overuse or imbalance injuries again. EVER! Over the last several years the only injuries I have suffered have been due to accidents. In addition, I seem to recover from accidents faster and I am more functional while injured. I try not to sit around, though. For me, inactivity is one of the worst things during recovery. If you get hurt and sit on your ass, you now have two problems to solve: get back in shape and recover any function you may have lost. Three days after my upper body was injured in the SUV accident, I was running again. Within a week I replaced my bike. And, since I couldn't climb, I put 1,200 miles on my new road bike within a few weeks. When it was time to get back to climbing, I only had that to worry about.

My food plan is as simple as it gets: keep the carbohydrates complex, eat poly- or monounsaturated fats, and keep the protein intake plentiful. Aside from that, a multivitamin takes care of the rest. The only things that vary are the proportion of carbs to protein (depending on training cycle) and the number of calories taken in (also varies with training cycle). As far as supplements are concerned, I take a protein powder post-workout, a multivitamin, and the occasional sports drink to rehydrate during my workout.

I have many rituals, but in summary:

I like routines and I like numbers. I keep everything on a timer and a log. Workouts, workloads, and rest times are all quantified, monitored, and recorded when necessary.

I never, ever, quit strength training throughout the year, though I do modify the routine as training priorities change.

No matter how much work I have piled up, I always reserve one day of the week to do whatever the hell I feel like doing, which is usually playing on tall rocks.

Last and by no means *least* is Ariel Ries. Ariel was raised in the Midwest cornfields by grizzly bears I tell you! "What?" "Screw you; we do have bears in Illinois. Where do you think the Chicago Bears got their name, huh?" Sorry, slight editorial dispute there. Anyway, as I was saying, Ariel is a force to be reckoned with. Since I've known her, she has always held a skate shop down, been an amazing artist and craftswoman, and a coordinator and does it all while flying down a hill at several miles per hour. A close cousin of skateboarding and luge, going down a concrete hill at the point of "you can't just hop off" is a serious game. Longboarders put in work. There is nothing like the good ol' feeling of speed wobbles and road rash to start your day.

Ariel knows that feeling and is a trooper. One of the kindest women around, she is also one of the toughest. Real easy on the eyes too fellas, so try to contain yourselves, as she is not clothed in her featured photo.

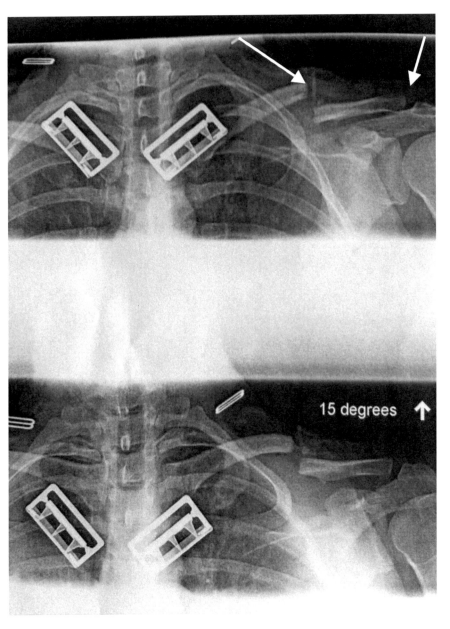

Photo: Courtesy of Ariel Ries

ARIEL RIES

"Ain't nothin' to it, but to do it." —Sesame Street

29

LONGBOARDER / SHOP OWNER

14 YEARS BOARDING

HOMETOWN: CARY, IL

CURRENT LOCATION: DEKALB, IL

I've owned a small town skateboard shop in Dekalb, Illinois since 2007 and I have been on the search for hills to bomb since I was 13 years old. I am a huge longboard and skateboard enthusiast and I love dancing, snowboarding, snow skating, and working out. My life revolves around skateboards. I sell skateboards, ride skateboards, promote skateboarding, organize skateboard competitions, demos, and lessons, and I even make art and jewelry out of broken skateboards.

I consider myself at 100 percent when it comes to my health right now, even though I technically have a bone that is forever broken in half in my body. As an "action athlete," I am always training and conditioning my body to be ready for physical activity. As far as my mental health goes, I feel as if it is directly correlated to my physical health. If I can't go out and sweat and do the things I love, then I go crazy.

My injuries have been pretty minor (knock on wood) and the worst thing that happened to me was breaking my collar bone and getting a concussion at the end of the summer in 2010. I broke my own rules when it came to longboarding. The rules are: no skating in an unfamiliar area after dark, wear safety gear when reaching speeds over 25 mph, and make sure the end of the run gives you time to make a proper stop. I broke all three of these rules and therefore broke a bone in half. *Snap*!

I hit a little gravel and my board flew from underneath me and I landed on my head. I felt a sudden pain in my shoulder and I stood up and yelled to my friends. As soon as they ran back to me, I said out loud, "I just broke my collar bone and got a concussion" like my body knew it before I even did. Immediately after spitting those words out I remember my body collapsing; when I opened my eyes, I was laying on the ground looking up at the sky and trees. I was straight tripping! I saw color-changing geometric shapes just dancing and moving around, and I thought to myself, "It's go time." I stood up and tried to walk and immediately blacked out and woke up again on the ground. Seconds later when I came to, I called my friend and he helped me get up and to the car and we drove to the emergency room. When I got to the emergency room, they did a CAT scan, an X-ray, and some other tests, gave me a sling, and confirmed what I had innately already known: I broke my clavicle and had a concussion.

A day later, I had a doctor's appointment and she gave me a brace that looked like a figure eight that went over my shoulders, under my arm pits, and connected between my shoulder blades. This was supposed to bring my broken bone together so it would connect. After seven weeks of following the doctor's orders, always wearing my sling and my brace, not lifting my arm, and taking it super easy, she took my X-ray and the bone still had not connected. **She told me that I had what they called a "non-union" break and that my bone would never connect on its own.** She gave me the option to have surgery, but since I didn't have health insurance, she said that I would be fine without it. I have full range of motion, but if I were to have a really bad fall, there is a chance that the broken bone will pop through my skin, which means immediate surgery. When I found this out, I had to make a decision: go into $10,000 or more of debt for a surgery, or keep on keepin' on, which I decided to do since I could completely move my arm and I really felt no pain. I looked all over the Internet to try to find out information on non-union breaks and the long-term effects, and I basically found nothing.

At this point, it's over a year later I don't let it stop me from living the life I love. I can still feel a dull pressure in my shoulder, but it's not painful. Since it's a newer injury, I really don't know what to expect. I have been focusing on conditioning and strength training my arms and upper body since my injury. I feel like if the muscles and tissue around the broken bone are strong, then the chances of it getting re-injured are less likely. However, I don't know if this is true. I did not take any supplements, pain killers, or prescriptions. I followed doctor's orders and still did not heal. My real coping mechanism has been to not think about it and to not let it stop me or scare me away from living.

I have to do something that makes me sweat every day. That's my number one rule. I try to switch it up all the time. You can't just do the same workout every day or you won't see results. I skate, go to the gym, hike, swim, climb, bike, snowboard, snow skate, hang from monkey bars—you name it, I probably do it because I love being active! As far as my diet goes, I don't limit myself. I eat whatever I want when I want, but I just try to keep my portions small and eat frequently. Luckily I enjoy healthier foods and I try to stay conscious of calories and ingredients. I feel like high-fructose corn syrup and convenience foods are an epidemic and I try to stay away from them.

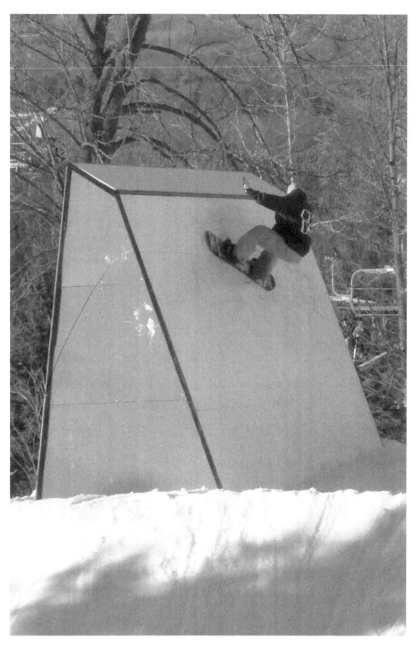

Ray Lang   Photo: Marjie Lang

3

MAKES SENSE TO ME

The health professionals in this chapter are the shit. When I first started to write *Tough Like You,* many people advised me to find medical professionals to legitimize the book. With good intentions, but misunderstood, they didn't realize that the content required no approval. The stories and recounts contain many references to hospital visits, medical procedures, physician advice, and treatments. Avoiding the hypothetical "what ifs," we were fortunate enough to have plenty "this is what happened" in the last chapter.

I chose instead to focus on areas of conditioning, prevention, and recovery. Coming from a slightly different angle than traditional Western medicine—which largely consists of "identify, stabilize and medicate"—these individuals are all passionate about atment, healing, conditioning, rehabilitation, nutrition, and using the body itself to either prevent or recover from injury and breakdown. They are *perfect* choices.

It's a no brainer. As mentioned in many of my articles previously written for *Focus Skate Magazine*, if you hear a "crack" you should be heading to the nearest hospital. Fractures can come with many other problems, especially when close to vital organs.

Common sense and the ultimate goal of the writings, which is getting to know *your* body, is the gauge at which a person decides to seek professional help.

Having an orthopedic surgeon write about bone surgeries for this chapter frankly would have been a little boring. Although vital in the recovery for many of the athletes featured, the basics of treatment would be redundant and the details much too specific and best left for medical journals.

Let's take a look at some advice and expertise from those that have chosen careers in helping us be more than we ever thought we could be, instead of just surviving.

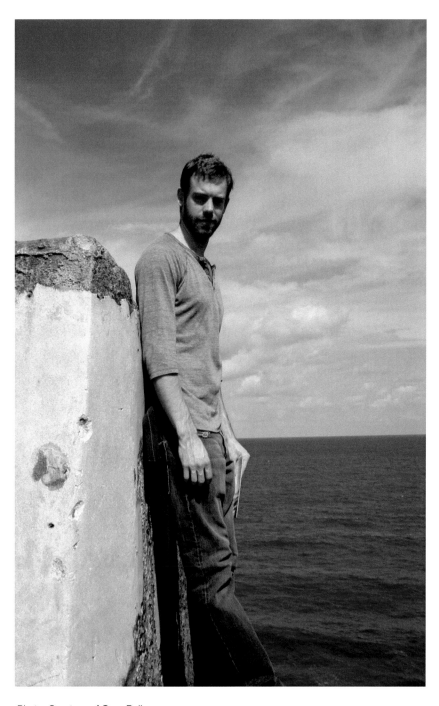

Photo: Courtesy of Greg Bell

GREG BELL

BODYWORK THERAPY

ACUPUNCTURIST

HOMETOWN: HILLIARD, OHIO

CURRENT LOCATION: CHICAGO, IL

The work I do as an acupuncturist and herbalist attracts all sorts of patients. Young and old, male and female, active and sedentary, patients with diagnoses from A to Z are all equally likely to show up at an acupuncturist's clinic in hopes that they will find the relief that other therapies did not provide. However, because I also specialize in Asian Body Therapy, particularly Tui Na and Thai bodywork, I have been seeing a growing number of athletes in my practice. These people need more than a gentle relaxation massage at their local spa, although there is a place for that as well. They need a more specialized and methodical, indeed a more clinical, form of bodywork. I combine this type of therapy with the benefits of acupuncture and herbal medicine to give these athletes an edge.

Nevertheless, there is a great deal of dietary, lifestyle, and self-care methods that can empower athletes to stay in peak physical condition. So when I heard that Amos was writing a book on this very topic, I was eager to contribute. I've made an effort to keep the following information straightforward and practical, with tips on how to prevent and heal injuries as well as enhance and maintain performance. As a physically active person in my own right, I have first-hand experience with all of this information and have included only that which has been beneficial for me and/or my patients. I hope it helps others as well.

Self-care for Injuries

Injuries are an inevitability for any athlete, and although there are ways of reducing the frequency and severity of injuries, it is crucial to know how best to nurse your wounds. Properly caring for injuries not only gets you back to the sport you love faster, but also guards against similar trauma in the future.

Minor cuts and scrapes are pretty self-explanatory, so I won't say much about that stuff. To the other extreme, broken bones will require a hospital visit, and if you need a cast, there won't be a whole lot of self-care you can do until it comes off. Most of the info I'm giving here applies to sprains and strains, and there *is* a difference. A sprain is a tear in a ligament, which attaches bone to bone—for example, an inversion sprain (aka a rolled ankle). A strain is a tear in muscle and/or tendon, which attaches muscle to the bone—for example, groin or hamstring pulls. I'll explain the importance of that difference later. If the sprain or strain is severe enough, you may need surgery, so it's important to get it checked out at the hospital, especially if you feel any instability in the affected joint. Self-care starts with determining which of the three stages (acute, sub-acute, chronic) your injury is in. Each stage has its own set of signs and symptoms and therefore, its own self-care protocol.

Acute:

This stage usually lasts for the first 2–3 days after injury, although it is more important to assess an injury based on the symptoms than the time frame. Depending on how the injury is cared for, the acute stage could last 18 hours or seven days. It is characterized by relatively severe pain, swelling, redness, and heat. Obviously, depending on the severity of the injury, this would be the time for a hospital visit, and I imagine that action athletes develop a pretty keen sense for when this is necessary. But unless you need a cast or surgery, much of the healing will be in your own hands.

The acute and sub-acute stages are the most important in terms of self-care because, just as a person's early childhood determines much of their later development, the care given to a new injury determines how it heals over time. Traditionally, experts have used the RICE protocol for acute injuries, but this method has come under criticism lately by some who are recommending the relatively new MEAT protocol. I believe the marriage of both gets the best results. More on that later.

RICE stands for Rest, Ice, Compression, and Elevation. This protocol focuses on reducing swelling, the idea being that in acute injuries, the body tends to go overboard with the inflammatory response and the swelling causes more damage to the initial injury. Rest implies limiting movement of the injured area. Ice and compression are applied to limit blood flow, and elevating the injured area above the level of the heart helps to drain excess fluid to reduce swelling.

MEAT stands for Movement, Exercise, Analgesics, and Treatments. The idea here is to promote movement and blood circulation in cases where there is injury to tissues with relatively limited blood supply and therefore, slower rates of healing. Movement and exercise encourage blood circulation to the injured area and ensure that fibrous tissues heal in the proper alignment. I will describe some specific exercises later.

Analgesics refer to the use of pain medicines. This is not necessary for healing the injury and is only intended to make the athlete more comfortable, so using them is totally up to you. Personally, I hardly ever use analgesics. Even when I was in the hospital for a kidney stone, I refused pain killers simply because, as hard as it is to bear, pain gives us valuable information about what's going on with our bodies. This is particularly true for musculoskeletal injuries. If you do choose to use pain killers, DO NOT TAKE ANTI-INFLAMMATORY DRUGS. A temporary, controlled, local reduction of inflammation may be necessary, but anti-inflammatory meds cause a systemic, prolonged inhibition of the body's healing response which is not desirable here. Finally, seeking treatments such as physiotherapy, acupuncture, ultrasound, and others is highly recommended.

Proponents of the MEAT protocol claim that RICE is only appropriate for injuries to tissues with a high blood supply such as the muscles. This is particularly important in the case of a blunt trauma to a muscle because individual muscles and groups of muscles are wrapped in fibrous connective tissue called fascia. Particularly in the lower leg and thigh, the fascia can enclose whole muscle groups in a compartment, which will not allow enough room for the swelling caused by a forceful impact. The compartment may build up with pressure from the excess blood and fluid, thereby cutting off the flow of fresh blood to the area and effectively starving the muscles to death. Once they're dead, they're gone for good.

On the other hand, for injuries involving the ligaments, which have little or no direct blood supply, there is a greater need for local inflammation to heal the injury. Also, movement of the injured area is crucial for healing ligament damage because this helps the collagen fibers to line up in proper orientation along the lines of tension. Without movement, the fibers of the ligament may heal in a jagged or crisscross orientation, resulting in a weak spot in the ligament that will be vulnerable to future injury. So, as the argument goes, the RICE protocol would only hinder the healing of a damaged ligament since it reduces local inflammation and limits movement.

It is important to note, however, that no reliable comparative studies of these two methods have yet been conducted to determine which is better. Many health professionals out there, myself included, have found that learning when and how to apply both systems together yields superior results.

During the acute phase, use RICE until the swelling and pain subside, which usually only takes 20–30 minutes. You can then remove the ice and begin doing some very slow, small, gentle movements of the area, being careful not to illicit significant pain. Do not use weight-bearing movements. Gradually, the swelling and pain will return and you will apply RICE again. Continue this process until a reduction of swelling and pain is maintained without RICE. You will then be in the sub-acute phase of the injury.

Sub-acute:

The sub-acute stage typically lasts for the next 1–2 weeks after the acute stage, depending on the severity of the injury. It is marked by a decrease in pain and swelling and an increase in range of motion. There still may be visible redness, bruising, or swelling and some pain with weight bearing. There are several self-care practices that are helpful here.

Movement of the injured area becomes particularly important in this phase when you're dealing with ligament damage such as a sprain because collagen formation spikes during this time, and you want these tissues to heal in the correct alignment. You should be testing your range of motion and doing some light stretching and massage. For injuries such as a sprained ankle or wrist, you can try writing the alphabet with the affected limb. As I said before, try to avoid eliciting pain with these movements, and avoid weight-bearing activities if they cause pain.

Contrast therapy is the alternation of hot and cold compresses on the affected area. The application of cold causes the blood vessels to constrict, thereby flushing out old, stagnant blood and inflammatory debris. Applying heat accelerates the metabolism of the affected tissues and dilates the blood vessels, bringing in fresh blood and healing factors.

By alternating the two, you can produce a kind of pumping action, much like ringing out a dirty rag, which speeds up healing by improving microcirculation and stimulating growth and repair.

The easiest way to do this is usually to take a hot bath and periodically remove the injured area from the water to apply ice. The ice commonly produces the desired effect within 30–60 seconds while the hot water will take about three minutes. Continue alternating hot and cold for 30–40 minutes and be sure to end the session with a cold compress to avoid swelling. This should be repeated daily for the duration of the sub-acute phase. If you do not have a bathtub or the use of a bathtub is not convenient for the location of the injury, you'll have to use hot and cold compresses. Make sure you use a moist heat compress as dry heat usually doesn't penetrate deep enough.

This is also an important time to include some kind of treatment from a sports medicine specialist as their expertise, skills, and resources can make a big difference in recovery. The more severe the injury is, the more urgent such treatments become. Physical therapists can provide you with a tailored exercise routine to ensure that the injury heals properly. A skilled practitioner of Chinese medicine can usually get excellent results by combining acupuncture with time-tested herbal therapies.

Most acupuncture clinics keep some traditional herbal liniments (topical medications) on hand specifically for musculoskeletal injuries. This may seem like a ridiculous suggestion, but the proof is in the pudding. I continue to see results with two liniments in particular: *Zheng Gu Xue* and *Dit Da Jiao*. *Zheng Gu Xue* is used in the treatment of hairline fractures and sprains, and I have had several people tell me how astounded their doctor was at the rate of their recovery, not knowing that the patient had been using *Zheng Gu Xue* religiously. *Dit Da Jiao* is an age-old remedy used by martial artists in the treatment of bruises and sore muscles. These liniments should be thoroughly massaged into the affected area at least five times per day especially during the sub-acute phase. You can also soak a first-aid wrap in the liniment for additional exposure. Your local acupuncturist can probably sell you such liniments, or, if you live in a big city, you can find them in Chinatown.

Chronic:

The duration of the chronic stage varies greatly and will depend on the type and severity of the injury as well as the care given in the earlier stages. It could last months or years. If the injury has been healing well, you may only be experiencing some mild weakness. Range of motion should be normal, and weight-bearing will cause little or no pain. Movement and exercise should continue, now with the use of resistance and strength training. A physiotherapist can teach you exercises that help you develop greater fine-tuned movement and coordination. If the injury did not heal well, you may still have some low-grade pain that is brought on by exercise or by moving in a certain way, and there may be a greater sense of weakness or restricted movement. If this is the case, you must see a sports medicine therapist, or the injury may never fully heal and you could experience continual re-injury.

It is important to note that not all injuries follow these three stages as I have described them here. Everyone is different and every injury is different. The last time I sprained my ankle about four years ago, there was significant swelling and severe pain to the point where I was afraid I might have broken something. I used RICE for the first evening and by the next morning the symptoms were gone and I was able to walk normally as though nothing ever happened. I still followed up with some exercises for strength and dexterity during the next week, but I haven't had another sprain since. Wouldn't it be nice if all injuries healed so well!

Self-care for Injury Prevention & Performance Enhancement

In Chinese medicine, taking preventative measures is considered superior therapy. By developing methods and habits that keep you healthy and prevent injury, you can become your own superior physician. Nobody knows your body as well as you, and when you fully get in touch with your body, you can not only prevent severe injuries, but also amplify your performance and overall health beyond your own expectations. Here are some of the recommendations I often give to my patients as a starting point. However, there is always room for improvement, and I encourage athletes to do their own research and to think critically and creatively about their health.

Warm-up exercises: It's common knowledge that you should warm-up before exercise, but not every athlete knows how to properly warm-up. Start off with 5–10 minutes of simple movements such as joint rotations. This is very important to avoid sprained ankles and the like. You can then move on to some form of light exercise; exactly what kind is up to you, but it should be adequate enough to raise your heart rate and warm up the muscles. End your warm-up with some stretching and be sure to focus on the parts of the body you use most in your sport. It's a good idea to consult a sports medicine professional on how best to stretch, because there are certain types of stretches that are safer and more effective than others.

The Epsom salt bath: Epsom salt (magnesium sulfate) is one of the great forgotten remedies; it's effective, versatile, and inexpensive. I always recommend this to patients when I do any deep manual therapy with them, as it prevents excessive soreness after this kind of work. The two components of Epsom salt are magnesium, a vital, yet undervalued nutrient, and sulfur, which is beneficial for joint health. In my experience, taking a warm Epsom salt bath before or after exercise can greatly relieve muscle tension and soreness. Magnesium from the bath has been shown to enter the bloodstream, where it acts as a muscle relaxant and mild sedative. Taking an Epsom salt bath before bedtime promotes deep, restful sleep, which is crucial for recovery from physical stress. For optimal effectiveness, most people need at least two pounds of salt in the bath water; soak for 30–40 minutes. I do not recommend more than three Epsom salt baths per week.

Develop and maintain healthy muscle tissue: This is one of the most important maintenance practices for athletes, and I have found most athletes to be shockingly oblivious to this information! Mainstream media has us thinking that tight, chiseled muscles are healthy. Sorry for the disillusionment, but this is simply false. Healthy muscle tissue should be loose and supple when not in use. In fact, you should be able to push your hand into a muscle and feel the bone underneath. If a muscle is already partially contracted before you use it, it will have less contractile force when you need to use it. In other words, a chronically contracted (shortened) muscle is weaker than it looks, hence the equation, length equals strength.

If the muscles feel like they are contracted even though they're not, you have unhealthy muscle tissue, because that contraction is stagnating blood flow, resulting in a slight but chronic starvation of the muscle cells. This causes sore or tender muscles, which brings us to another point. Because muscles have relatively few pain receptors, they should not be painful to press on. If a muscle is painful with palpation, it is a sign of inflammation due to chronic contraction and stagnation of blood flow. Of course, we're all walking around with painful, tight muscles somewhere in our bodies. It is simply the result of wear and tear from the various activities of daily living, but that doesn't mean we shouldn't try to maintain healthier muscles, and, for the action athlete, it can have a huge impact on performance.

So how does one keep their muscles healthy? Maintaining a regular stretch routine is very important to keep muscles at their normal length. As I mentioned earlier, athletes should work with a physical therapist or personal trainer to develop a stretch routine that fits their needs. If you have the financial means, the best thing you could do for your muscles is to get a weekly massage from a skilled massage therapist or body worker. However, taking regular Epsom salt baths offers you a convenient time to do some self-massage. With the muscles relaxed in the warm bath water, you can make much better progress. First, spend some time just feeling the muscles in different parts of the body. Get familiar with the intricacies of the muscles, the different layers, and where the muscles attach to bone.

With enough practice, you can start to feel the fibers of the muscles. Massage them by running your thumb, fingers, or elbow down the length of the muscles going with the direction of the fibers. You'll want to use enough pressure so that it is tender but not excruciating. Do not expect the muscles to completely change overnight, but eventually you will notice your muscles feeling spongy and yielding under pressure. You want the change to happen gradually, and it will take time to develop the palpation skills. But with time and practice, you can develop an invaluable skill to prevent injury and heighten performance.

Learn to rest when you need it: This seems to be one of the biggest problems I have when working with athletes. When I ask them to take a couple of days off from their sport or exercise so their body can heal, they refuse to do it. Indeed, they often seem addicted to exercise! If you are feeling tired and achy, try taking a day or two to rest and see how you feel afterward. This also applies to a pro athlete who is preparing for a competition. It is better to rest and recover your strength than to push yourself too far and compete in a state of exhaustion. If you are recovering from a cold or flu, it is extremely important to avoid strenuous activity until you are fully recovered.

Another important point is to make sure you are getting adequate sleep. For the action athlete, it is crucial to get plenty of deep sleep. Taking cat naps is refreshing for the mind, but it takes more time for brainwave patterns to slow down enough for deep sleep, which is necessary for the body to recover from physical stress. If you are suffering from insomnia or are not feeling rested when you wake, seek help from a health care practitioner.

A word of caution for female athletes: if you experience a diminished menstrual flow or the cessation of your period altogether, this may be a sign that you are overexerting yourself. While men have a relatively steady flow of energy, women have more of an ebb and flow to their level of energy due to the menstrual cycle. Their bodies spend part of the month building up blood and energy, and when the period starts, that blood and energy are expelled from the body. This means that during and right after the period, women are more vulnerable to fatigue. If your periods stop or become very light, your body may be desperately trying to conserve energy, and you should take it as a sign to start resting more.

Inflammation and the diet: Diet is another area that must be addressed if an athlete hopes to optimize performance and overall health. The specifics of diet and nutrition for athletes are better left to a certified dietitian. However, as a health-oriented man who has done a lot of research and experimentation with my own diet, I can give some general tips that you may not hear elsewhere.

Many of the health problems we face in a modernized society stem from years of an inflammatory diet. Refined sugars and other processed foods tend to be pro-inflammatory and lack the complete nutrients they had before processing. Dairy tends to be very inflammatory and, contrary to popular belief, is not necessary for healthy bones. Traditionally in China, dairy is rarely, if ever, consumed and yet their rates of osteoporosis are lower than in the U.S. where dairy is a staple. In my opinion, the bulk of a person's diet should consist of fresh produce. Small portions of meat are essential for athletes, as they have much higher protein demands than most people. Supplement your Omega-3 intake with fish oil or flax seed oil to maintain joint health.

Hypnosis: This one is especially important for pro athletes. Many of the greatest athletes in history, including Michael Jordan, worked with hypnotists for performance enhancement. It is pretty common knowledge that mental visualization of a routine or exercise improves one's efficiency when actually physically performing it. The same areas of the brain are activated whether you are thinking about the activity or doing it. Hypnosis augments this phenomenon. With a little background info on your sport and your specific routine, a skilled hypnotist can take you through the routine step-by-step and help you prepare mentally for a competition or other milestone.

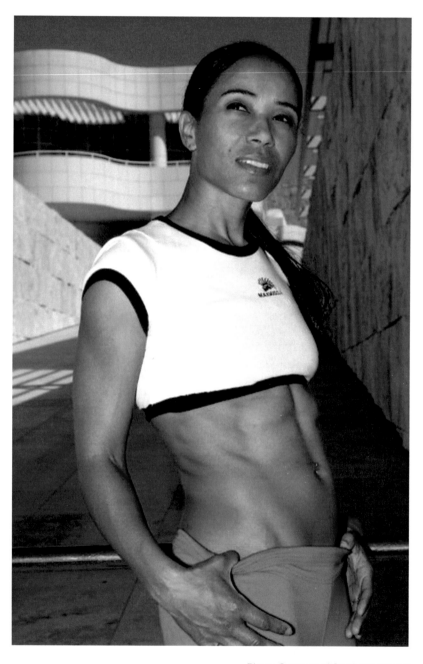

Photo: Courtesy of Stephanie Person

STEPHANIE PERSON

PERSONAL TRAINER

SKATEBOARDER

HOMETOWN: LOS ANGELES, CA

CURRENT LOCATION: LOS ANGELES, CA

Inception

My story started in 1984 when a friend of mine let me borrow a skateboard that she found. After having the board for two weeks, I was freaking out. I wanted a board as a gift for my upcoming birthday. My mother said, "Stephanie, it's your 17th birthday; you're turning into a woman. What do you want? I'll get you anything you want within reason." I told her I wanted a skateboard. She said, "You're joking," and I said, "Uh no. I want a skateboard." She tried to persuade me to get a dress and offered to buy me any clothing I wanted but I insisted that I wanted a skateboard. She finally agreed and we went down to a skate shop to pick up a board.

My first board was a Tony Hawk. The guys at the shop told me that they went skateboarding after closing the shop and I could skate with them but *only* if I could keep up. I took a 30-minute bus ride to get there and I *did* keep up. The first day, we skated all over a part of downtown in Los Gatos and I was killin' it. The guys were amazed and continued to invite me to roll with them.

One of them mentioned an amateur league I should join called the Castle League. They offered to sponsor me because it was a requirement for entering the competitions. From there, things started to connect.

There was a girl in my English class who always wore custom *Thrasher Magazine* shirts. They weren't retail and were specially made with graphics all over the place. It used to bug the hell outta me that this girl didn't skate and had these dope *Thrasher* shirts on. It turned out her boyfriend was an older guy who put on regular skateboard competitions; it's actually the one you see in the Powell *Future Primitive* video. At the competition, the girl and I talked and I found out her boyfriend was also friends with all the guys at *Thrasher*. We sat next to each other in class and I was invited to join them at one of the next competitions.

My mother told me I couldn't go. That was the *first and only* time I ever snuck out of the house and went away for the weekend. I jumped in their car at 5:00 a.m. and headed to Sacramento. When we got there, there were 20 people in an apartment with everyone all over the floor and just one chair in the room. I sat in the chair because there was no place to lie down. Tommy Guerrero was there and offered me a spot near him. I didn't know who he was at the time. The next day, everyone was divided up into cars and of course I didn't have a car. The girl and her boyfriend had left so I had to fend for myself. I hung out with Eddie Reategui, Christian Hosoi, and Christian's dad. I'll never forget sitting in the car with Christian and his dad; Christian kept calling his dad "bro." I thought that was pretty weird.

Another time, I found myself in the company of Bob Schmeltzer and Per Welinder, two freestylers who had just done stunt work for the *Back to the Future* films. They were going to an Upland competition. Through mutual contacts, I was fortunate enough to go with them. We drove to Upland Skate Park and me, being a naïve girl, saw a skinny kid sitting on his board, padding up, and Bob says, "Hey Tony! How you doing?" I was like, "Damn, that's the guy on my skateboard!"

Those two sequences of events put me right in the middle of the professional skateboard scene and then a third event tied it altogether.

I put on a street skateboard competition during my last year in high school in 1984. I called a bunch of sponsors with my pitch. When I told them I was a girl and putting it on by myself, they thought that was pretty cool and they said, "Sure! We'll sponsor your event." I was living in San Jose at the time, which was smack in the core of skateboarding's growth.

The competition went well. Over 800 people a lot of famous skateboarders came to the competition. One of them was Corey O'Brien who told me that the event was amazing and said, "Let's put on a pro competition." There used to be a competition near Santa Cruz called the Capitola Classics. He said, "All the pros have nothing to do after this so why don't we just grab them from one event and do a backyard, underground, quick throw down competition at the Montegue banks." So we did.

It was a huge competition. I was a little black girl running around with the judges and doing paperwork. Tony Hawk was there. Everyone was there; you name the pro, they were there.

People would ask, "Who's putting on this competition?" and others would say, "That black girl over there!" That was the beginning of my life as a skater and it eventually brought me to where I am right now.

I entered a lot of California amateur competitions. I started with street, then graduated to ramps, and eventually skated vert predominately. At one of the street competitions I met a lot of Europeans and they said, "You should come over to Europe." So I did.

I was set to leave in April and return exactly four months from the day I left. However, right before leaving, I got sponsored by Santa Cruz Skateboards. I made the cover of a newspaper doing a front side air over a 4 foot channel at Raging Waters Skate Park and the guys at Santa Cruz loved it. They invited me to do a demo with Rob Roskopp and Christian Hosio at a 49ers versus Bears playoff game at Candlestick Park. We did the halftime show and it was amazing. The ramp was 16 feet wide, metal and horrific, with 2 foot platforms with no hand railing ramp. But we did the demo and it was *sweet*.

I finally went to Europe and met loads of people; it was amazing. I mean *a-ma-zing*! I was young, free, and had no responsibility. I went back a second time after that and Santa Cruz covered the trip. The second time I went, I stayed for almost 16 years. I left the U.S. at 19 and stayed in Europe until I was 35.

Overseas as a teenager I toured, did competitions, was on television, went to art shows, hung out and life was great. But at some point, the party was going to end.

The skateboard shows and competitions were slowing down in the 90s. Skateboarding kind of hit a lull. I wasn't ready to come back home so I went to Denmark and realized how difficult it was to rent a place so moved to Sweden. I just hung out for what was supposed to be a short stay. I skated in a competition in Stockholm, Sweden and that's when my life changed.

The Awakening

In the competition, on my 26th birthday, I tore everything imaginable in my knee. After the injury, I had two choices: I could sink or swim. I decided to swim. If I wanted to recover and get over my injury quicker, then I needed to start asking questions and start reading.

Part of the complication with my knee was that it was infected. When you have an infection, you need to boost your immune system and fight bacteria, so I started reading about how to do these things and which foods to eat. But the real push came from a friend who said, "If you want to get the strength back in your leg, you should go to a gym because physical therapy is such a sick environment; it's sick for your mind and it's sick for your emotions." Working out gives you an overall growth hormone effect; if you lift your arm and do a bicep curl, you are essentially going to be releasing hormones that are going to affect your entire body…including a weakened leg.

Now I Get It!

When you walk into the gym, the first things that come to your mind are big traps, big shoulders, overdeveloped chests, and knuckleheads. But after being there for a couple of weeks, I realized that these people actually knew a lot about physiology, biology, kinesiology, and nutrition—it was amazing. That pushed me further into wanting to learn more about the entire body: how to build muscle, how to recover, and ultimately, how to get my legs back on track. I still had it in my mind that I would get back to skate competitions and also start skiing soon (which never happened), but when the skateboarding door shut, another door opened: the incredible world of the human body.

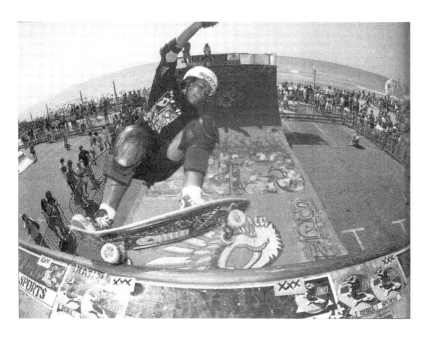

Stephanie Person (Circa 1990)

The Body

You have many different systems in your body. If you're an athlete, just on a superficial level, it's about a mind-to-body, mind-to-muscle connection. A motor-unit recruitment is a reaction in the muscle—when you think of something and then you make a muscle group do something, by repetitive movement, your body grows more units of muscles and those muscles are learning what to do. That's called muscle memory. There are systems that contribute to being a good action sport athlete. It's all about the core. It holds you in positions, keeps you from falling, and keeps you in contorted positions.

Once you subconsciously figure out the mind-to-body connection, which is essentially your core, you can then start to become more aware and begin to manipulate your body. I think when you start doing a sport like skateboarding, you don't understand what's happening mechanically on an analytical level. It's all subconscious. You feel it and you do it; it's all a feeling. When I skateboard today, post-injury, I think everything out and visualize the movement before I do it. It can be really fascinating and can also suck because it takes away the spontaneity to actually have to think before doing the trick or movement.

We have different systems—musculature, hormones, adrenal, brain, and the repair and recovery system. With my clients and with skaters especially, people who do extreme sports are constantly putting themselves in a state of catabolism, which breaks down and tears the muscle. A person is either getting sore or overusing their muscles, which results in micro-tears in the muscle.

My suggestion for athletes is to never overtrain because at that point of overuse, it takes a long time to heal, causing your body to produce too much cortisol. Cortisol is your fight-or-flight hormone which makes you run from danger like from a saber-tooth tiger. Having an adrenaline rush, coupled with cortisol, causes gluconeogenesis. That is your body's ability to break down muscle tissue in order to give you that rocket fuel to run away faster from danger. But that hormone in excess is toxic. They actually call cortisol the "fat-storing hormone" because you constantly break down and teach your body to store fat in case of an emergency, so you can be able to have the energy to survive.

Basically your body is in survival mode. It doesn't matter if you're running from a saber-tooth tiger or running from a board at your head or if you're just trying to stay on your board. Your body goes into the fight-or-flight mode and tells itself to "get quick energy to the muscle and brain as soon as possible." That's what's going on when you do a crazy run on a big vert ramp: your body is trying to produce energy. If the energy is going on for too long of a stint, then your body will go into a catabolic phase. A lot of body-builders lift too much weight. It's counterintuitive—you're building, but you're tearing down your body at the exact same time. If you're young, it's okay because your body has a quicker repair system than someone who's older. Someone 40 years old who goes through the same type of workout doesn't produce recovery cells as quickly as they could when they were younger.

But even if you're younger, you still have to think about the catabolic effect. You can later develop osteoarthritis, arthritis in the joint, and injuries that take you out of the game. Also, if you skate, BMX, or surf without good nutrition, your performance will be affected. Not enough proper nutrition affects your thyroid, which controls your metabolism. Another thing that can be affected is your adrenal system. Adrenaline can be used to wake you up in the morning and it can also be released quickly if you're doing a sport. Binding globulin hormones affect how much testosterone or estrogen you're producing, which is needed to keep up your musculature. Overtraining and eating improper foods will mess up all those systems. When you're younger, you can recover quicker but when you get older, you will literally look in the mirror and age.

Sleeping patterns are also important. During prime sleeping hours, especially during 10p.m. and 4 a.m., your body is slowing down. That means the blood is getting thick, your heart rate is slowing down, and you're essentially hibernating; now your body can start to repair damaged cells. You can't sleep during the day and have the same effect because there's another aspect called your circadian rhythm. That's a really important system to understand because that affects your hormones.

When the sun goes down, you have receptors in your eyes that can sense the light diminishing, which tells your body to produce more melatonin (a sleeping hormone) and less adrenaline. Adrenaline is released very slowly through your system to keep you awake and alert and when your body is ready to sleep, it needs to slow down because it needs to shut down and repair; melatonin is then released in small increments. Then you fall asleep and your body goes into repair mode. If you have an all-night job, your body can't repair. It's in a false sense of feeling awake and overproduces adrenaline the entire day. This has a serious catabolic effect because adrenaline in excess, along with cortisol, gives you a quick amount of energy that you don't need. That puts stress on your thyroid which controls the way your body burns calories.

The reason why it is important to understand these systems is because it's the difference between being an elite athlete who can last for years and elite athlete who burns out really quickly and develops an injury. If you don't have enough energy and you go skate in a pool and you're hypoglycemic because you didn't eat enough of your carbohydrates, then you don't have enough energy and muscle contraction to do a five-hour skate.

Nutrition

I cannot believe how much we have been lied to about nutrition. Every time I'm around people, I hear things like, "No! I don't want to give up my carbohydrates!" It's so bizarre because if you say to people, "Would you eat the Teflon off a pan or would you put your head in a microwave? Would you drink coolant from your car?" People would be like, "Hell no." But essentially, it's kind of the same thing in the sense that carbohydrates are toxic.

Carbohydrates

Our bodies *can* metabolize and break down carbohydrates, but in tiny amounts. Our pancreas releases insulin, a hormone that carries blood sugar. Carbohydrates break it down into a molecule called glucose. Your body takes that out of the blood and to its destinations: your liver, muscles, and fat cells. Once it enters your liver, it becomes glycogen and then it is released in small increments back into the bloodstream. It's interesting that in starvation mode, your body will tear itself down in order to fuel the brain. That's why they say you can go days without food: your body will feed off itself. But you cannot go days without water.

Carbohydrates come in two forms: a complex and a simple carbohydrate. A complex carb is dense and the saliva cannot break it down in the digestive process. You may think a cracker is a complex carb because it starts from a grain and the grain starts out as complex, but then it is pulverized, bleached, and broken down and the grain becomes a simple carbohydrate. If you put that in your mouth, it will begin to liquefy and eventually empties into your small intestine. The small intestine has absorbable walls to carry nutrients, so your blood sugar rises at that point.

Eating a complex carb like broccoli is a whole 'nother thing. If you put broccoli in your mouth, it will just sit there for a long ass time. That's considered complex. Dense vegetables have a lot of fiber. Obviously if you eat too much fiber, you're not going to be digesting the nutrients to feed the body. Isn't that weird? We're always being told to eat fiber. But if you eat too much fiber, you're going to poop too much and you're not going to digest nutrients because those cell walls are so tough. That's why some raw foodists like to keep their heat under 160 degrees and cook food really quickly; that way, they break down some of the cell wall, keep the nutrients, and won't have so much cellulose in the system.

Starches

Bread, white potatoes, rice, and cereal are all starches. A starch molecule does not have, especially if you break it down, a lot of digestible fiber. When you eat a pulverized grain, you're left with the starch. It is like eating sugar. In fact, scientists say that a Snickers bar will have less sugar in it than a baked potato. That's because there are fat, butters, oils, and nuts in the Snickers bar, and anything fat will slow down the digestive system. Something that goes through your body too quickly peaks your blood sugar too fast. Glucose creates a glycation factor and that's when sugar becomes sticky and inflammatory. Your liver will convert that into a substance called triglycerides which is a fat that can cake, plaque, and do a lot of damage to the cells in excess. Unfortunately, our fruits and vegetables have been genetically modified. Our fruits especially, have been made to be more sweet; the genes have been spliced and we're not getting the fruits and vegetables we did a couple hundred years ago, if not a thousand years ago, when our systems became fully evolved. Sour berries, meat, and yams used to be a human's primary diet. The amazing thing about humans is that we're like scavengers: we can metabolize anything. But you have to realize that if you eat and drink coffee and processed foods which are nutrient deficient, you're not fueling your body with something that can repair cells. That's why I can look at people in the face and know that they have dysbiosis, an imbalance in the digestive system that causes inflammation of the bowels which shows up on the skin. It is caused primarily through sugar, but toxins, chemicals, and pesticides are also contributing factors.

So how does this all relate to being an athlete? *Everything relates* because you need tools to fix your cells in order to be a good athlete.

Fats

Fats are amazing. Our bodies are made up of a lot of fat. Our cell membranes, lungs, and brain, are made of fat. Even our sex hormones are modulated by fat intake. Fat is another source of energy that our bodies can use. If you want to be a good athlete and have a lot of testosterone (if you're a guy), you need to have enough fat in your system. Not only does fat affect the serotonin in your body which makes you feel balanced, but it also affects your sex hormones which have a lot to do with musculature and overall health.

Fats are separated by mono-, poly-, unsaturated, and trans fats. Poly-unsaturated fats include seed oils and vegetable oils. Monounsaturated fats consist of olive oil and nuts. Saturated fats are animal fats and coconut. Trans fats are hydrogenated vegetable fats. As an athlete, you need to be careful.

Science is astonishing. We have all of this great technology, yet we have more cases of cancer, auto-immune diseases, prescription drug deaths, and heart disease THAN EVER BEFORE. How can we be so advanced, have great low-fat diets, and still have so many cases of obesity and illness?

Nutrition in our world

In the 1930s, there was a dentist named Weston Price. He was curious about the teeth of people in different cultures and countries. He set out to look at other cultures and really wanted to go to the most remote places possible. He found very low cases of cavities, teeth and cranial malformations, disease, and cancer—all of these things that were a rising factor in the United States. Weston Price is pretty badass in my book. He did a lot of research, went all over the world and photographed people and their teeth; he heavily documented this concept. He found that cultures that didn't consume grains or eat low-level grains and ate more fat had fewer mouth and body diseases. About five years from now we'll be having a conversation saying, "How could we be so stupid?" Conventional doctors will be like, "Oops."

But people want their carbohydrates. The soy, wheat, and corn industry is a trillion dollar industry; it's not going anywhere. These industries and the Food and Drug Administration make more money than oil. People get sick with food and then they are handed drugs. When you look at commercials on television, it's no mistake—people don't pay for that advertising unless people are buying the product. There's a supply because there's a demand. If you turn on the television, you'll be inundated by pharmaceuticals. It's bizarre and I've noticed it within the last five years; all these crazy ass drugs people take and we've never been sicker before as we are now. It's just a matter of time.

The Inuit tribe, a native and indigenous tribe, eats whale blubber because the whale fat is very hard to digest. That's their primary source of nutrition. The Maasai tribe in East Africa drinks a lot of milk, which is high in calories. The Polynesians eat fish and a lot of coconuts, which are saturated fats. We may think these foods are bad for us, but these tribes are actually healthier because of fats!

We're now learning that saturated fats *don't* clog your arteries. Corn is a cheap source of food for cows which results in acidic meat (Meat is terrible. This is why vegetarians say, "See! Meat makes you sick!"). If you put hormones in your animals, like in eggs, chicken, and beef, all of the meat becomes pumped with garbage. Even the top soil, where vegetables grow, has been depleted. To grow a crop for a normal farmer years ago, you would plant the seeds and wait a few months for the soil to remineralize itself before you could plant again. But we're finding ways to plant again, over and over, resulting in mineral and nutrient-deficient plant-sourced foods. Not only do we have bad meat, but we have bad vegetables, hence all the cancer, disease and toxins, and pollution crap. Believe it or not, **this all affects your performance as an athlete.**

Cholesterol

We've learned that total cholesterol numbers are not an indicator of heart disease. The problem is if you have high levels of HDLs in comparison to LDLs. These are lipo-proteins that carry cholesterol to the cell. Cholesterol is actually a repair hormone that we produce in our own body.

Proteins

Proteins are made up of 20 essential amino acids. These are the building blocks of tissue repair. When you don't have amino acids, you start to suffer. This is connected to your sex hormones, which is connected to your adrenal system, and that is connected to your brain and heart cells—everything that builds tissue. Vegans have pretty tough bodies. It takes a while for the body to catastrophically catabolize. In the beginning, vegans feel high, they feel great, but over time they begin to develop issues they can't explain, like they can't heal as fast or they have a hard time reproducing, and so on. This affects your ability to excel as an athlete.

A question many people have is, "When should I take my proteins?" You should probably eat a post-protein meat source or whey protein as a way to replenish depleted sources of protein and amino acids that you need. You definitely need at least 60 grams, and as an athlete you'll want about 100 grams. Body-builders take in about 160–170 grams of protein a day and that's the amount of grams per body weight. Too much protein, in the absence of healthy fat, makes your body convert that into sugar, which ultimately gets converted into fat.

All these things have to do with keeping healthy cells, making you a badass athlete—fats, carbohydrates, proteins, and obviously a lot of vegetables and fruits are essential. Fruits and vegetables have macro-nutrients, flavonoids, and antioxidants that help boost your immune system.

Final thoughts

Stretching is important as an athlete. Athletes tend to get tight hamstrings which will snap the ACL. It can also tear other systems in your knees. It is really important to stretch your hamstrings and your lower back because your lower back is connected to your hamstrings. You need to be able to bend over and touch your toes without feeling pain. Stretching is essential for all athletes, no matter the sport. If you get tight muscles, you don't have joint mobility and you tend to develop a shorter range of motion which can create arthritis and injury, among other things. You need to strengthen your core (chest, abs, back, and lower back) especially in extreme sports. You don't want too much of an overdeveloped chest or back because you tend to put your weight forward if you have weak shoulders; an overdeveloped back will compensate for the balance in your chest. Same thing with your abs. You don't want overdeveloped abs and an underdeveloped back because then you will hunch forward and have a hard time stretching your lumbar back region.

Skate! Hydrate yourself! Lower those damn carbohydrates! Don't eat stupid protein and energy bars; they're garbage. A bottle of water is pretty much the same as tap water. In fact, bottled water is not as strictly regulated, so companies can put more shit in it and take the bad taste away. Get a filter; try to get a filter that actually takes away fluoride. As far as warming up goes, jog in place for one minute with one minute of recovery time; do this for five minutes, stretch, and then go workout. This will give you a nice, ample supply of blood to the muscle so you don't snap your ACL!

It is important to realize that your thoughts are connected to your hormones and your hormones are chemical. Your cells can actually become addicted to negative hormones!

Leptin is a hormone that can go out of wack. Your serotonin levels can also drop in the presence of too many carbohydrates. Eating too many carbohydrates can be attributed to autism, schizophrenia, bipolar disorder, and anxiety.

Coffee is very bad! It's processed and acidic. It puts stress on your adrenal system, pumps you up, freaks you out, and gets you amped. A lot of weight-lifters take a pre-workout caffeine supplement which slams the adrenal system. Your body is not meant to have your heart rate up like that. They *believe* it is a fat burner, but what other stress is it putting on your whole body?

Chill out! Have a good time! If you notice your heart rate is up because you're pissed for whatever reason, try to calm your shit down really fast because you're putting your body in a catabolic state and you'll develop stress hormones which ultimately make you suck as an athlete. Just take deep breaths. When I started skateboarding again after I injured my knee, I felt my heart bouncing out of my chest. I got my heart rate down because I knew that if I could get less adrenaline in my system, I was going to be more malleable, flexible, and calm during the skate session rather than having too much adrenaline, putting me in the context of injury.

Live hard, bike hard, skate hard, snowboard hard, and swim hard! Be more conscious of what you put into your body; be aware of your mental health and anxiety, and GET GOOD SLEEP between the right hours. If you think you're a night owl, you're lying to yourself. There's no such thing.

The only thing we exist by is the circadian rhythm: we're supposed to wake up at the crack of dawn and sleep when the sun goes down.

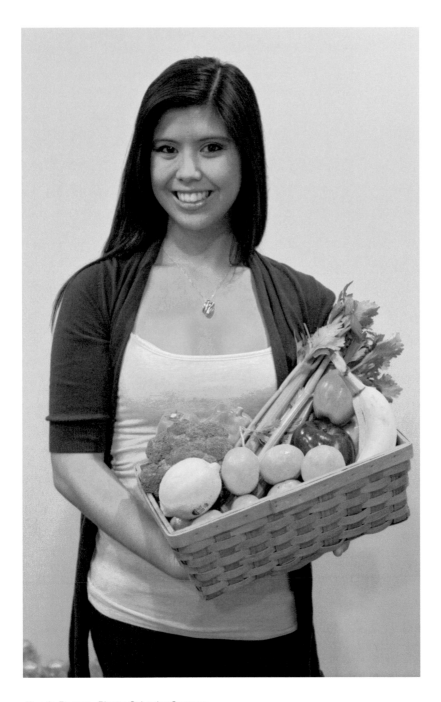

Krystle Ramos   Photo: Salvador Campos

KRYSTLE RAMOS

DIETICIAN

HOMETOWN: DARIEN, IL

CURRENT LOCATION: CHICAGO, IL

Hydration & Moderation

Hello! I'm Krystle Ramos, a registered and licensed dietitian. I believe water is the sweet elixir of life. It dictates how we feel as well as how well we perform. Often, sore muscles can be prevented by simply drinking enough water. Water is vital to your body. It composes up to 60 percent of your body weight, flushes toxins out of your system, and helps lubricate your joints and mucus membranes in your ears, nose, and throat. The Mayo Clinic recommends drinking two to three liters of water per day. That is just a little less than one gallon. In times of heavy perspiration, it is recommended that you increase your water intake to prevent dehydration.

What exactly defines dehydration? It is simply taking in less water than you are losing. Dehydration can be mild enough to cause discomfort or severe enough to cause death. Odds are, you have suffered mild dehydration once or twice in your life. Spending a few hours skating, biking, etc. in the summer sun and heat is a common cause of dehydration. Dehydration can easily be avoided by drinking plenty of water.

The best gauge of hydration is the color of your urine. The darker it is, the more dehydrated you are. If you are well hydrated, your urine should be a light, hay-colored yellow. Other signs of dehydration include sleepiness, dry mouth, headache, dry skin or lips, constipation, and thirst. If you see these signs in yourself, drinking a couple extra glasses of water or a sports drink like Gatorade should help bring you back to normal.

When you stop sweating even though you should be, you may be in trouble. The basic idea is to stay well enough hydrated to not get to this point. If your body stops sweating or if your sweat is more like sugar and salt crystals than sweat, you need to stop what you are doing and seriously consider seeing a doctor. If you or your body is against that, for whatever reason, make sure you get sugar, potassium, and sodium in you, as well as fluids. This is why sports drinks work. Orange juice mixed with an equal volume of water and a dash of salt can help. Grabbing a banana, some water, and having a few small, salted pretzels is another potential fix. It won't take much, but make sure you eat or drink slowly and wait a while before you continue on, especially if you choose not to seek medical help.

Protein is the building block of life, and is critical for building and repairing damaged muscle and body tissue, producing hormones, regulating body processes, contracting muscles, and transporting nutrients. Protein can also give your body stamina and energy. Most people in America, even vegetarians, eat enough protein on a daily basis. Protein is found in nuts, animal products, whole grain products, legumes, hummus, cheese, leafy green vegetables, and soy products, just to name a few. When selecting protein sources, leaner is better. Choose meats cooked without oil, leaner cuts of meat, low fat dairy, fish, or poultry whenever possible.

Carbohydrates, sometimes called carbs, are your body's primary source of fuel. They are easily digested and great for quick bursts of energy, but without protein or fat, that energy will not last. Carbohydrates are found in any grain (rice, bulgar, couscous, bread, corn etc.), fruit, any product with sugar (sometimes called fructose, dextrose, lactose, sucrose, mostly any ingredient that ends in "ose"), most dairy products, starchy vegetables (potatoes, corn, acorn squash, butternut squash, spaghetti squash), and legumes (garbanzo, pinto, kidney and white beans, lima beans, dried beans, such as black-eyed, split yellow, and green peas; and miso). Complex carbohydrates are better choices; they supply more nutrients than simple carbohydrates. Whole grains and high fiber foods, such as raw fruits and vegetables with their skins, are examples of complex carbohydrates. These are the carbohydrates that will give you more sustainable energy.

A healthy diet will include some fat. The healthy fats your body needs are called monounsaturated fats, polyunsaturated fats, and omega fatty acids. These fats are found in olive oil, walnuts, nut oil, sunflower seeds, avocado, and cold water fish, such as salmon. Many food products are now enriched with omega-3 fatty acids.

Now that we know a little background on the macronutrients (protein, carbohydrate, and fat), how do we tie it altogether? You do this through well-balanced meals and snacks. The icon for healthy eating has changed recently. They all essentially portray the same information, focusing on reasonable portion sizes, vegetables, whole grains, etc. My personal favorite is a plate illustration from The University of Michigan, called "The Great Plate."

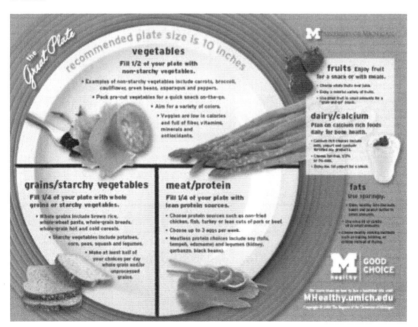

This image is my favorite because it is very easy to use and understand; it encourages meals as well as snacks. Meals should be eaten off a 10-inch plate, which is fairly standard. It encourages half of the plate to have bold, bright, colorful vegetables like broccoli, carrots, tomatoes, green beans, peppers, or leafy greens. These vegetables should be prepared with little or no fat. The vegetables that will offer you the most nutrients (vitamins and minerals) are the ones with the boldest colors. The more colorful the vegetables on your plate are, the more variety of nutrients you will receive. About one quarter of your plate should be starchy foods, such as whole grain breads, brown rice, or oats. The emphasis here is on complex carbohydrates. The last quarter of your plate should have protein foods like lean meats, eggs, and non-animal based proteins such as edamame, tofu, temphe, garbanzo beans, hummus, kidney beans, and other soy or legume based foods.

What about fruits and dairy you ask? They are also on "The Great Plate." Dairy is important because it is one of the richest sources of calcium. Fruits are important because like vegetables, they offer a myriad of nutrients (again, go for colors!). They can be incorporated in healthy meals as components of salads or beverages, or used as stand alone foods and beverages. A small bowl of berries and milk (or a milk substitute for those of you who abstain from lactose or true dairy products) can be a delicious and healthy dessert. These items can also be a great snack.

What about junk food? It's *junk* food. It fills you with empty calories, generally adding unnecessary and unhealthy fats, sugar, and sodium to your body. They void your body of nutrients.

Soda actually strips your bones of calcium. It's a poor choice to fuel your body, especially if you want to participate in your sport for long periods of time.

Does this mean you should never eat cakes, cookies, chips, or candy? No, but it means you should do so in moderation and make sure your diet is very healthy otherwise. By that I mean that the overwhelming majority of your meals and snacks, at least 80 percent to 90 percent of everything you eat and drink, is nutrient-dense and super healthy. A small candy bar, cookie, or small serving of chips once or twice a week is not going to hurt you or highly impact your health or performance; it just has to be kept in moderation. A small serving is less than a handful! And once or twice a week *means* once or twice a week!

How do you eat healthy on the go? Plan ahead and know how to make healthy choices at convenience stores or wherever you stop to grab a quick snack. I longboard, mostly to commute across the city, and LOVE skating up and down the lakefront or through the city just for fun. I get hungry every few hours and can never drink enough water on a long skate. I pack healthy snacks and water in my backpack whenever I can and if I can't or forget, I run to a store. Either way, I choose low-sugar, high-fiber granola bars, dried fruits (or fresh fruits if they won't get crushed in my bag), nuts, and whole grain crackers. If the weather allows, I will pack a sandwich; peanut butter and banana tends to hold up well when I'm out and active. On a very hot and humid day, I will grab a sports drink. I choose fresher fruits, low fat items, complex carbohydrates, and lean proteins. This works for me!

Miriam Zmiewski-Angelova   Photo: Stoyan Angelov

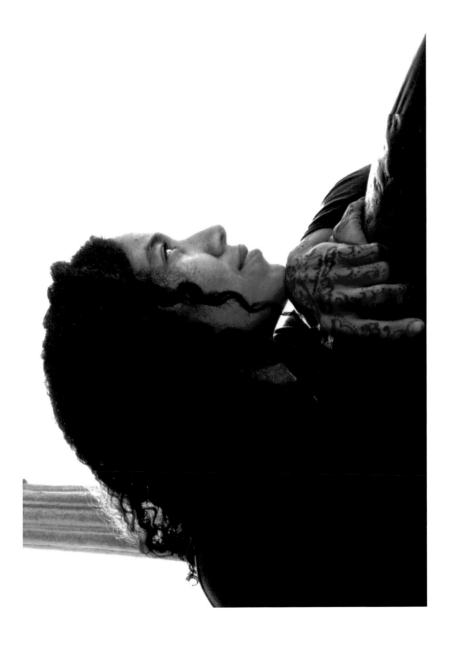

MIRIAM ZMIEWSKI-ANGELOVA

PUBLIC HEALTH

HOMETOWN: CHICAGO, IL / TAIPEI, TAIWAN

CURRENT LOCATION: TUCSON, ARIZONA

Public Health and Wellness Through Action Sports

My name is Miriam and I received my formal training in public health, received my master's degree in maternal and child health with an emphasis in Native American community health and wellness, and am a registered trainer of A.S.I.S.T: Applied Suicide Intervention Skills Training. I spent the first seven years of my life in Taipei, Taiwan while my father worked on his residency in naprapathic medicine. I then bounced around for about a decade: to Chicago, some international locations, and finally onto Tucson.

When I think back to my adolescent years, I remember watching my stepfather (the author) in our front yard practicing his tricks on one of his many seasoned boards plastered in a collage of stickers.

When he gave me my own board, I primarily coasted along the street and attempted some small tricks. I personally never graduated to any noteworthy skating street or on a half-pipe, but I enjoyed being part of the skater crowd. Seeing my friends and family having fun was always motivating. It was also cool to say that my dad was a skater. To this day, whenever I visit Chicago, a city of three million and counting, I am guaranteed to eventually find him at Wilson Skate Park in the late afternoons and evenings. Furthermore, his help in coordinating the skate demos and kid clinics at Lollapalooza and Kidzapalooza spoke volumes about the application of skateboarding and action sports in general for youth development programs.

A Brief Introduction to Arizona's Vibrate

Native Skateboard Culture

My life and work thus far has been diverse, eclectic, memorable, and fulfilling. I am Choctaw, Cherokee, Fond du Lac Ojibwe, African-American, and Ashkenazi. I am also the founder and president of 7G Consulting LLC, a company that develops innovative methods of promoting culturally-relevant, community-driven and strength-based life-skills development programming for Native youth and their communities. Over the past four years I have lived and worked in Arizona as a public health professional on various Native American youth and family health, wellness, and empowerment programs. I have also had an opportunity to provide assistance and instruction as a suicide intervention skills trainer in various locations throughout Arizona within several tribal reservation communities and in Colorado. In each of these settings, the community members and youth I met have shared their strategies for coping with stress, trauma, grief, and loss and ways they are promoting health and wellness within their community.

In the past two years, there have been some really amazing projects in and around Tucson focusing on community health and wellness, and developing innovative methods for getting youth outside and active. In the summer of 2009–2010, I worked as a training consultant and co-instructor with several remarkable individuals at a handful of Native youth leadership camps throughout the Tohono O'odham nation. Together, we developed several culturally relevant programs and activities around life-skills development and healthy coping skills for youth.

Through the Tohono Land Connections (TLC) summer program, the G.R.O.W. N.A.T.I.V.E. project, and the Native Education Alliance, I worked with Carmella Kahn-Thornbrugh (*Navajo*), Casey Kahn-Thornbrugh (*Mashpee Wampanoag*), and Melodie Lopez (*Hopi*) in teaching youth about preserving their cultural traditions around planting and healthy development. The youth also connected the benefits to eating healthy, increased energy, endurance, and performance. Juanita "Cheryl" Green (*Mashpee*

Wampanoag), Director of the Tohono O'odham Nation's Youth Suicide Prevention – Youth Leadership Camp asked me to help develop programs that focused on ways that youth can sublimate feelings of stress, anger, sadness, and grief with physical activity, music, art, and writing. We found that several of the youth were interested in skating or currently skated and show skateboarding helped them deal with difficult situations and connect with their peers.

In November of 2011, Lisa Falk of the Arizona State Museum and renowned artist Ryan Huna Smith (*Chemehuevi/Navajo*) partnered to develop a spectacular health and wellness event entitled, "Through the Eyes of the Eagle." The event promoted, "It's up 2 U," a comic book featuring the adventures of three young Native skaters who learn about the importance of eating healthy for diabetes prevention. "It's up 2 U" has been made into an app that delivers the message of health, wellness, and skateboarding using methods that speak to our tech-savvy generation. In addition to the comic book and app was the debut of Ryan's beautifully designed skateboard that was showcased, along with others, bearing the names and designs of Todd Harding (*Creek*), Dustinn Craig (*White Mountain Apache*), Douglas Miles (*San Carlos Apache/Akimel O'odham*), and Walt Pourier (*Oglala Lakota*). In an interview about the Native skateboard culture, Todd Harding stated, "Native skateboarders have been putting culturally significant designs on skateboard decks almost from the beginning. The expression is unique, and something (he) doesn't see among other cultural groups." (Briggs, 2009)

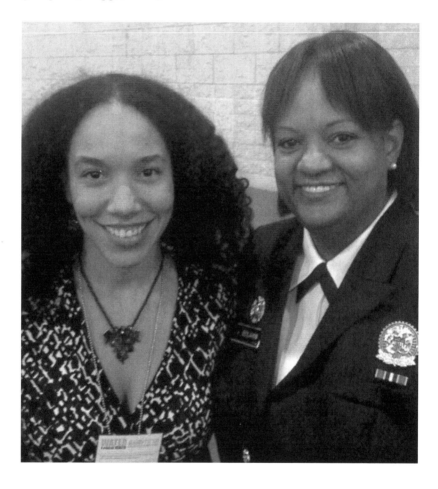

Miriam with Surgeon General Dr. Regina M. Benjamin at the 2009 APHA Conference. The American Public Health Association is the oldest, largest, and most diverse organization of public health professionals in the world.

Skateboarding: An Embodiment of Independence

The sport of skateboarding embodies the spirit of independence. It is independent and offers the rider a thrilling, challenging, and goal-oriented activity that does not necessarily require a group for participation. Skateboarding also provides a convenient means of transportation, thus promoting a sense of self-reliance. **A desire for independence is a typical part of social and emotional development for adolescents, and with independence comes a need to have an individual identity** (Healthwise, 2010). As adolescents develop, they begin to substitute the support, advice, and identity initially provided by parents and family by that of their peers. The researchers at Healthwise.org (2010) also noted that adolescents attempt to express their individuality by mimicking the style of dress, mannerisms, and activities of their friends or older adolescent and adult role models.

Skate parks offer the opportunity for youth and adults of varying levels of skill, fitness, and socio-economic status to connect, interact, show off their talents, model proper technique, and encourage the use of personal safety equipment in a relatively safe environment away from traffic. Unfortunately, skate parks are not available in every community. The Tony Hawk Foundation (2012) estimated that there are only 3,000 skate parks to service the more than 9.3 million skateboarders nationwide, which means that the majority of skateboarding occurs in the streets and in busy public settings. The combination of the lack of access to safe places for children to play and increasing volumes of traffic in residential streets contribute to community disconnect and limits on children's freedom to move freely around their neighborhood for fear of motor vehicle-related injury (Thomson, 2009).

Skateboarding 101: Untapped Potential for School-based Physical Education Programs

"Quality physical education serves as the cornerstone of a comprehensive program because it provides the unique opportunity for students to obtain the knowledge and skills needed to establish and maintain physically active lifestyles throughout childhood and adolescence and into adulthood." (CDC, 2011)

Imagine for a moment that skateboarding was offered among the sports that students could participate in through school-based physical education programs. Skateboarding offers a unique opportunity to pursue a physical activity that teaches focus, goal-setting, and resiliency. It also encourages self-determination, builds self-esteem, creativity, and individuality, and doesn't suggest a standardized approach to the style of skating in order to achieve proficiency in the sport (Tony Hawk Foundation, 2012). Furthermore, the endorphins released during frequent, vigorous physical activity can help reduce unhealthy risk-taking behaviors and feelings of stress, hopelessness, and suicidality (Cash, 2007; CDC, 2008; Taliaferro, et al., 2008).

Physical activity and healthy eating are linked to an increase in life expectancy, quality of life, and the reduced risk of numerous chronic diseases (CDC, 2011). The U.S. Department of Health and Human Services (HHS) recommends that children and adolescents engage in either moderate or vigorous physical activity for a minimum of 60 minutes daily—something that is age appropriate, enjoyable, and offers variety. Additionally, three days within a given week should include activity that incorporates vigorous intensity, and strengthens muscle and bone (CDC, 2011). Information collected from various current and former skaters and various skateboarding resources report that this sport offers a variety of maneuvers and tricks that require vigorous intensity and can strengthen muscle and bone through continued participation and practice.

Resiliency, goal setting, and self-determination are critical elements in the development of healthy adolescents and are also among the characteristics of effective youth development programs as defined by the U.S. Department of Health and Human Services (Catalano, et al., 2004). The lack of standardization in skateboarding promotes freedom of expression, individuality, and allows for the inclusion and engagement of individuals with diverse backgrounds and abilities. Individuals are able to connect on a common, healthy interest and form bonds of friendship and support that can last a lifetime (Tony Hawk Foundation, 2012). These characteristics are also among those supported by the

Centers for Disease Control and Prevention report on school health guidelines for healthy eating and physical activity. *Guideline 4: Implement a comprehensive physical activity program with quality physical education as the cornerstone* (CDC, 2011). **By acknowledging the vital link between healthy adolescent development and the health-related behaviors they choose to develop, we offer the greatest opportunity for their transition into healthy adults** (CDC, 2003).

Action sports are not only a great way to stay physically active and develop friendships but can also offer the added benefit of sublimating harmful risk-taking behaviors and suicidal ideation.

A study by Taliaferro (et al., 2008) examined the suicide risk in high school youth and the protection afforded through physical activity and sports participation. Their findings revealed a reduced risk of hopelessness and suicidality in males who took part in frequent, vigorous activity. Participation in sports had a protective effect against hopelessness and suicidality in both males and females. To sublimate feelings of stress, anger, hopelessness, and suicidal ideation, some youth may seek out risky behaviors. Cash (2007) recommends "providing students with alternatives for healthy risk taking, rather than attempting to eliminate risk taking entirely. Taking safe, supervised, strenuous physical activity, such as skateboarding, running, or working out, can release natural endorphins that meet adolescents' need to take risks." By providing skateboarding in a school-based setting, students can learn skills needed to promote safety and reduce their risk of suicide, violence, and unintentional injuries throughout their lives (CDC, 2008).

My hope for the future of skateboarding is a greater appreciation of action sports and wider acceptance of the benefits and applications in educational settings.

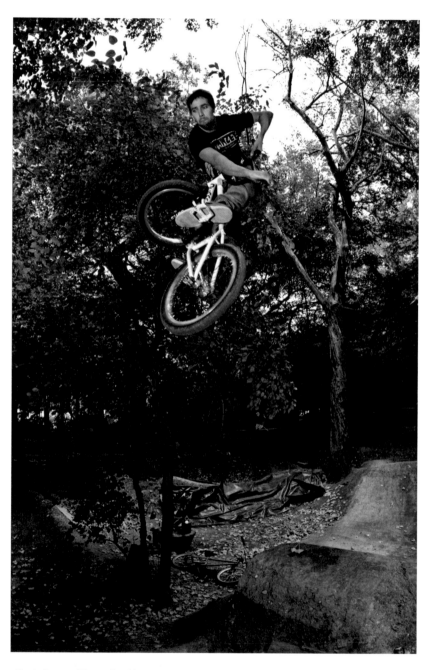

Kevin Porter   Photo: David Leep

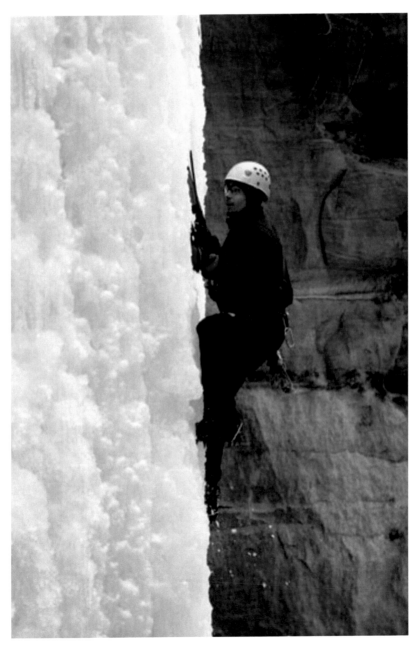

Stoyan Angelov   Photo: Miriam Angelova

4

"It impresses me that I still enjoy this thing. It's like this endless bounty that I haven't seemed to deplete yet."

—Jesse Neuhaus

Tough Like Me

Hi. I am a 45-year-old skateboarder, senior writer for *Focus East Coast Skateboard Magazine* out of Philadelphia, and team manager for a successful Midwest skateboard company with a very talented team called Character Skateboards. I am also the author of *Tough Like You.*

For close to two decades, I've had a great passion for learning all I could in the world of health and healing. Somewhere along the line I started to fuse skating, healing, and avoiding injury into published articles for skateboarders. Almost immediately, early teen skaters and seasoned veterans were asking questions and commenting on the articles. Skaters are a tough crowd. Successfully getting them to take a minute and think about anatomy, nutrition, and alternative methods of healing was quite a surprise. I had found ways to incorporate health into the minds of some of the most physically talented individuals on earth.

My story of injury, conditioning, and longevity featured here is slightly different from my fellow athletes but follows the same theme of learning to adapt, overcome, relearn, and strengthen oneself.

My life as a skateboarder started out in a small area of Chicago called Jeffery Manor. I remember the neighborhood being ethnically mixed: black, white, and Hispanic. By the time I was 11, it was predominately black. That's Chicago for you. It was, and remains, a lower-class hood that had its problems but was always close-knit. It was the kind of place where you would get into fights but usually knew who was about to punch you in the face and either confronted or avoided those situations. I would imagine it's the same now except that a punch could easily be a gunshot. Times change.

As a child, my friends and I played everything from organized little league to basketball, tag, and tackle, to "run and scream like idiots" across the neighbor's lawn who we knew was going to yell at us. We had a lot of games and they were fun as hell.

However, all that changed late '70s when we got a hold of skateboards. Not only were we playing harder, but now we had a mission—a mission that didn't end after each game or fantasy but was "game on" all summer long.

I wonder what the working-class people in the neighborhood must have thought about us preteen, little black boys that had found our *own* something creative to occupy our days—something that had absolutely *nothing* to do with the neighborhood programs, local playgrounds, or any former athletic activities.

My friends and I spent hours skating. We made a route along the sidewalks spanning five row houses. The houses had oval walkways that extended from the main sidewalk up to the doors. We created a skate game called "SkunkBelly." The object was to skate close together as fast as we could, avoiding collisions, and maneuvering much like racecars on a track. The only difference here was that SkunkBelly involved inevitable contact.

With integrity and some ethics, our mission was to strategically line ourselves up behind someone, at least a sidewalk square away, and shoot our board out and into the back of theirs while screaming "SkunkBelly!" No joke! We played this game for years. Mind you, at that time we were skating smaller and lighter plastic Free

Former, Fiber-Flex and Banana Boards. Like a torpedo launch, you had to be directly behind and not too close to your victim. There were other rules too, like you couldn't "skunk" during a turn or when someone was gaining speed after a fall. Another component of the game was to constantly gain more and more speed as it went on. We learned to weave, cut, and power slide like crazy to avoid letting someone lock onto you as a target.

It sounds dangerous, but I don't recall any serious injuries. Usually the most that would happen was bailing like crazy when your board was struck, or the often fun pile-up, and stumbling into everyone else. The worst of course was being the recipient of a perfectly zeroed "SkunkBelly!" shot and "wilsoning" out.

Those were the days—days long before anyone would ever call me Soma.

I never set out to be "Soma." In fact I always thought it was kind of weird when people gave themselves aliases. It was in a high school English class when a friend yelled out, "Hey that's your name backwards!" We were reading *Brave New World* by Aldous Huxley. Soma was the "ideal pleasure drug" that kept society from feeling pain or unhappiness.

My initial thought was, "Cool, my name backwards is the shit." It wasn't until a decade later that I started to use it for my music production company, then skating and writing, and it eventually became what I was called. I also learned many other meanings for it and felt it was fitting.

I was Chicago-born Amos Stephen Fuller in 1966. My parents later falsified my birth certificate so I could start school early. Because of this, I spent my school days as the youngest in my classes. My parents worked hard to send me and my sister to the best schools in our area. I was lucky enough to have gone to the same grade school for eight years and then to a prestigious high school for four years. My high school was an all-boys school known for producing college-bound men, often successful despite environmental influences. We got paddled and occasionally slapped!

I credit my teachings, both academic and disciplinary, as a big factor in saving my ass later on in life and wouldn't change a thing about my childhood. I traveled the U.S. with my parents and although we weren't well off by any means, we saw and experienced a lot. I was exposed to various parts of the world, especially the good, and knew right from wrong. Everywhere we went, I wanted to take my board along.

I did go on to college and before finishing school, went to the military. My days were just starting to get gnarly. I was out to live life, and life itself was my action sport.

With such a solid upbringing, having supportive parents, education, talents, and resources, it must have thrown those around me off a bit when I became a homeless addict.

It definitely surprised me! After all, I was the early grade school kid amazed by the human body, and carried my older sister's biology book around and studied it—that same kid that taught himself aviation by reading books and was eventually given the opportunity to co-pilot a small plane when his father paid for a plane ride on a vacation. Funny how life can change. Like a good friend recently said, "You never know what the average person on the street has been through." I'm lucky to be alive.

It's fairly easy writing about myself *now*. My story could be a whole other book in itself, but with details omitted, I will stick to relevant experiences. It's been over 12 years without any alcohol or substances in me; it's just a recount of a time past and gone. Although gone, not a day goes by where I don't think about where I've been. Skateboarding was a major player in my new life over a decade ago.

I remember spending a year as an inpatient in rehab. Even then, I thought about skateboarding and the feeling of moving fast on a skateboard. The thought alone calmed my very electric body; I constantly yearned to feel the sensation. Somewhere during the process of relearning to sleep through the night and my neurotransmitters relearning how and when to secrete dopamine and serotonin, my psyche adjusted to *no* narcotics.

This was a very difficult time. It took my body six months before I could sleep without night sweats, anxiety, awaking, and discomfort. Talk about a slam and fall! I had screwed things up pretty badly.

Before that time, skating was just something I did. I always had a board and rode when I could. Much like music, it was just there since childhood.

I never knew skateboarding had become a part of who I was and certainly had no idea it would become one of the most important things in my life, only second to my children, family, and few other things.

The transition from then to now was not easy. It involved a lot of *tough* not just from me, but from those around me as well. Before my decade-long downward spiral, I was married with a beautiful wife, daughter, and newborn son. My story was not a street story. I made self-destructive choices at a time when things were good. I had a self-employed functional family, luxury station wagon and sedan in the driveway, a personal recording studio, money, and all other things people dream about.

During and after the spiral, along with my health, those things went away. Again, fortunately for me, I had learned a bit about the body, got healing techniques from my wife, did self-motivated research, and was raised with some morals and common sense.

Armed with prior teachings and an open mind, *things changed.* Even as I write now, I find myself in front of my computer in my beautiful, industrial loft home with a pine music stage in my living room that my amazing band practices on, and a phone full of numbers of both family and loved ones. I have a glass of 100 percent natural juice to my right, a wall of class photos of students I have taught for the last eight years, walled skateboards for collecting, and also what I personally consider to be art. In or outside of my home, I'm surrounded by inspirational and talented people and things.

Lessons learned, I wouldn't wish addiction on my worst enemy. It's a slow, painful deterioration of mind, body, and soul. Addiction can leave deep scars and very few resurface from its depths. I am, as of today, one of the fortunate ones. Like a Chinese finger trap, it's easy to get into and hard to get out. Athletes in general have to pay special care not to develop a dependency on substances. Painkillers, such as Vicodin, work well during injuries but come with a hardy habit to break when taken for prolonged periods of time. All in all, what feels good is not always good for you.

When I emerged back into the real world over a decade ago, I instinctively felt the drive to heal. Although clean from substances, I needed to move fast and *feel* life. For me and many other action athletes, it's natural to have a restless desire to experience and be reassured that, "I'm alive." This doesn't exactly equate with what most people would call an "adrenaline junky." I think it has more to do with knowing that like a child, you're still learning and growing. We have a need for perpetual momentum.

Throughout history, many cultures, spiritualities, philosophies, and individuals have embraced the concept of the "inner child." The child within each of us is ultimately creative, alive, energetic, and simplified. It is our unconditioned "true self," shaped prior to social fears, stressors, and influences.

That secret portal allows us to capture our true nature and free ourselves, even if only temporarily, from life's woes in search of serenity, like that of an innocent child's mind—the ability to be as simple as possible while simultaneously visualizing the impossible. My thoughts, feelings, and actions are all mine and no one can ever take that away.

Somehow, those beliefs *have* internalized themselves for me and I credit them as also being another major part of who I am today.

At 45 years old, I'm fine and I am healthy. I have been riding a skateboard for over 30 years. It has become more natural for me to skate than walk. It feels weird to walk sometimes, as if the board is supposed to be under my feet at all times, even if I'm just going from point A to B.

I don't skate to stay fit. I skate because I enjoy the personal benefits and the culture. Ironically, for losing a decade of any real progression experienced in darker days, I don't feel like I'm making up for lost time or trying to stay young.

I naturally feel younger as time goes on. My injuries heal the same as my fellow skaters in their early 20s, and luckily I *haven't* found myself saying, "Oh man, I'm getting old" *too* many times. Granted, I didn't spend my 20s and 30s flinging myself down stairs like many other skaters my age with legitimate complaints, but I *have* started to fling myself down stairs *now*. **Despite what most people believe, you *do* still have a skeleton after 40 and your bones can be fortified to do just about whatever you want.** I have frequent sessions by myself in downtown Chicago. My ankles, knees, and everything else land down on the concrete (or the board) hundreds of times a week. From two to seven feet in the air at high speed and impact, it's a regular way of life. I feel fine. Sore sometimes, but fine.

I can imagine non-skaters seeing me and thinking, "That dude is having a mid-life crisis." It's actually quite the opposite, though. I'm on a mission to skate; that's it. From that comes growth through constant challenges, ideas, and infinite possibilities, so I guess I am in fact literally *growing* old, with an emphasis on growing. I'm not just *getting* old. It feels better this way. It feels healthy.

My skateboarding injuries include a torn ACL early on, a broken foot, toe, and wrist; a smashed lip that split to the teeth,; a thumb that needs a tendon reconnected; and several ankle sprains. They have all healed except the thumb tendon. It requires surgery one of these days. My right knee has chronic patella discomfort but nothing debilitating.

Another injury includes a confused nervous system due to methamphetamine, cocaine, and opiate use for years. I take mild epilepsy medication to help adjust my nervous system along with natural holistic practices. At one point, I went through extensive year-long testing because physicians suspected I had Multiple Sclerosis, but it was ruled out. During one test, dye was injected into my bloodstream and an ultrasound was used over my entire body. The doctor performing the test was happy to let me know that I had the least amount of arterial plaque that he had ever seen in someone over 25 years old; I was well over 30 at the time. I am truly blessed to have gone through addiction without any related disease like hepatitis or other things that hang around and slowly kill you.

Life injuries, such as broken relationships with family and other things have all healed or are healing too. Like a broken bone, some fused together stronger than before the break.

My regiment includes daily flaxseed or fish oils (EFAs), coral calcium, Ester-C, derived from calcium, a vitamin I've found to be much more effective and beneficial than regular C; milk thistle; and a few other herbs I've taken regularly for years. I am also a fan of MSM, a sulfur supplement that naturally occurs in our bodies, but is often lacked due to modern diet. MSM is directly responsible for joint, tissue, tendons, and muscle health and has been shown to help in the healing process when part of a regular supplement regimen. Research it for yourself. The EFAs I also take daily do wonders. I have great skin—seriously. Not that I'm hyped about my skin, but it is really soft and resilient. It heals very fast and leaves few marks. I contribute that solely to flax and fish oils that I have taken daily for the past 10 years.

Don't get me wrong. I'm not saying I won't wake up tomorrow with pancreatic cancer or something. I do the best I can to try to prevent those types of ailments by using remedies such as milk thistle, a proven liver cleanser. Inevitably though, at some point, something is going to break down in our bodies. We're mortal. Hence one of the main reasons I prefaced the book with not being concerned about how long you live but *how* you live, which in turn does affect longevity.

I stretch and meditate using a combination of various techniques and positions, taking bits and pieces from yoga, Toltec meditation, traditional prayer, and whatever else I have found useful to *my* body and mind. I've found one of the best techniques is morning in-bed stretches. Before rising, I spend a few minutes drawing the ABC's with my toes and ankles, extending everything to its furthest point. This has proven to be an invaluable habit. I notice a huge difference in the way I feel throughout the day by stretching before I'm actually up. I also continue to touch toes, slowly aware of each vertebra's reaction to my stretch. Moving around throughout the day is crucial, especially for people working a desk job, staring at a screen for hours. Rotating your hips and head frequently throughout the day provides flexibility. It's a really amazing little thing to do. With feet comfortably spread apart and hands on your hips, slowly rotate clockwise in a circular motion about 20 times and then do the same counter-clockwise. Keeping your feet in place, this stretching exercise loosens your lower back, hip joints, knees, and surprisingly, your ankles quite a bit. The hip rotations also help with digestion, as the colon itself is virtually massaged during the process. Hip rotations look weird to people if you're in public but fuck 'em.

I've noticed people are having a harder time getting around. They walk funny, are cumbersome, and stiff. Boarding a bus and taking a few steps up is difficult for the majority of people I observe. I see more and more people with limps and are hunched over—I'm talking young and old. Statistically, we all know there is quite a bit more obesity. They even called it an "epidemic." I believe there is more arthritis and joint discomfort in people than ever before too. I didn't do the research on that, but I don't have to; I've been watching humans for 45 years and can tell the difference. It really hit me after getting rid of my car a year ago and taking public transportation more. Even young professionals came in one of two categories: those that looked like they were active and those that didn't. It was *that* noticeable.

It seems that like the common cold virus, we must take preventative measures just to maintain health. It's as if people these days *have to* workout in some way to combat inevitable obesity and unhealthiness due to processed foods, stress, apathy, and a slew of other toxic factors in life. People ask me if I work out and I tell them no. Maybe one day I will but I'm not a big fan of gyms. Running on treadmills while watching the news doesn't do it for me and however politically incorrect this may be, beautiful women in exercise pants *is* a distraction! I could easily see myself dropping a dumbbell on my foot, not focusing on what I should be doing. Regardless of my opinion, the benefit of weight-training is evident. I know skaters that lift and they have a very powerful style, but it's not for me.

I enjoy my three S's: skateboarding, swimming, and soccer. The latter two I rarely practice, but my upper body stays toned because it's always in use. The cardio from skating burns fat and the stretching helps my upper body muscles define themselves through everyday activities. I recently bought a heavy punching bag again and have my own version of martial arts that I practice. With a little help from growing up with a martial artist and a fondness for the teachings of Bruce Lee's *Jeet Kune Do*, I think I do fairly well. My favorite exercise is actually using the bag with my eyes closed. I will spar with the 100-pound bag swinging back and forth in the darkness for a good hour sometimes. No real reason, but I do think it helps with balance. I have to constantly adjust my position in relation to the bag's returning direction and that's after I make contact with it, not being able to see.

I've been told I have a great body and should develop my chest more. Blah! Why? I'm not a body-builder! I respect the hell out of body-builders *but I'm not one*. The comment was made simply in relation to appearance. I'm a *skate rat* at heart. I have enough clothing to open a shop, but will often wear the same pants for days because they feel good. I sit on curbs, sweat all summer, dry and sweat more, and use a shoestring as a belt. It's complicated and most wouldn't understand. Many real skaters care little about their appearance but naturally look good from the intense physical nature of the activity. The bottom line is that we leave home every day, knowing there's a chance we'll be dirty, sweaty, and sometimes bloody. Shoes that we skate in don't stay pretty and no matter how nice your latest LRG shirt might be, it's gonna come in contact with the ground at some point if you skate or bike. Having this lifestyle entails a certain amount of humbleness and realness. Appearance is not high on the priority list for most. However, *bathing* most definitely should be and is! A shower or bath after a day of rippin' is an action athlete's best friend, often revealing the sting of scrapes and burns you didn't even realize you had gotten that day.

The fashion industry knows. They have been borrowing from action athletes' styles from the beginning. Long before hipsters were wearing flannel shirts, skaters and bikers were. That list goes on and on so I won't even go there. It is a good thing that many of the companies are owned by us now.

Anyway, back on track! My diet consists of very little gluten or dairy. I consume lots of rice products including rice milk, rice bread, and rice pasta, and no caffeine. I do eat a hell of a lot of cookies, though. I am not a purist and truly believe we all are different and different things work for each of us. However, I have learned to be open and listen to those that study what makes us be the best we can be, especially health consultants like the ones featured in *Tough Like You.* They not only know what they're talking about, but they know things that more practically relate to everyday life.

I also consume quite a bit of tobacco. Hmm. A book on health and healing written by a dude that smoked the whole time he was writing? Yep. Now would be a good time to either get the point of *Tough Like You* or toss this book out the window. Hopefully you continue to read on.

One thing I set out to do when writing, and feel it has been successfully achieved, was to connect realistically with my readers. Even the accounts of the past are in relation to the now. This body of work is for the human that is, and will always be, a work-in-progress.

We all have imperfections. Once identified, we now have the choice of dealing with them or not. If you're obese, a book can't make you thinner. If you have anxiety, reading a chapter on stopping anxiety attacks won't make them go away. However, reading facts, teachings, and experiences of others *can* inspire and expose you to that which fuels change.

We all have injuries of one form or another and we all instinctually have the desire to heal them. On many levels, healing should be an academic standard that all children are taught, along with math, science, and reading. It's an impeccable part of what makes us survive. As tough as we are, we are also extremely fragile. Most realize this too late in life and find getting older a very hard thing to do.

I suggest continuing to proactively learn and live, not with an inundated mind, but rather the clarity of a child. Continue to GROW.

I'll keep skating with the best of them, learning a new trick every year, and when my body says "stop," I will.

But probably not.

If you want to experience all of the successes and pleasures in life, you have to be willing to accept all the pain and failure that comes with it."

—Mat Hoffman

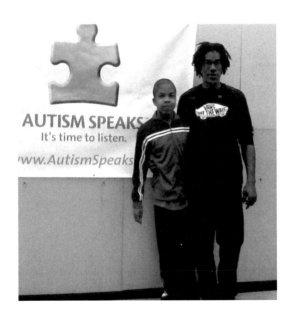

Amos Soma Fuller with son, Artist, at Chicago's
Annual 2011 Autism Speaks - Walk for Autism.

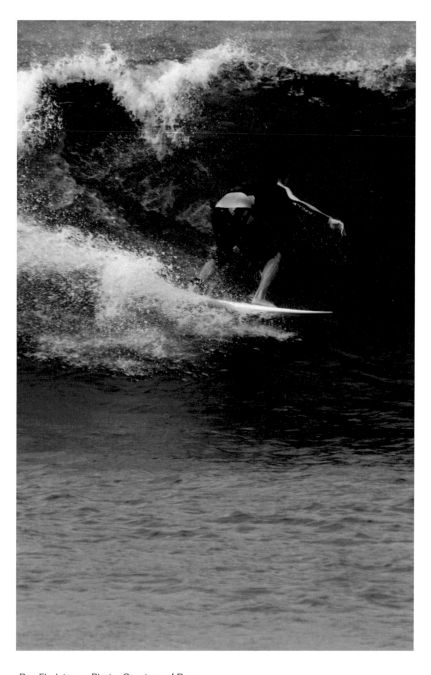

Rex Flodstrom   Photo: Courtesy of Rex

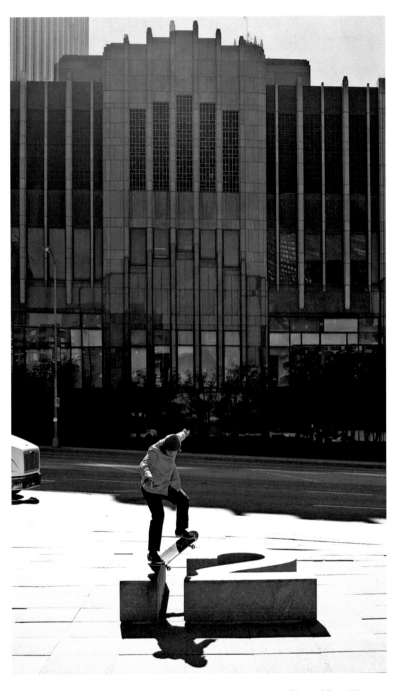

Justin Luu   Photo: Miguel Huerta

5

BACK SIDE NOTES

A few things I didn't have a chapter for, but thought you might find interesting:

- Most action athletes have decent posture. I think being aware of our posture is a good habit. Eventually, it will become an unconscious body awareness that will help us to stay in tune with our physical self as a whole.

- Freezing water or sports drinks on warm days not only provide you with hydration, but also cool you and last longer as the liquid slowly melts.

- I think we can all agree that feet are important. It's well worth the time and effort to find shoes that work best for *you*. Style is one thing, but support, cushioning, ventilation, and wear are ultimately the deciding factors in what shoes work best for you and what you're doing.

- I drink rice milk, or rice drink, whatever you want to call it. There is much controversy and misconceptions concerning dairy. Is it good for you or is it a contributing factor to many of the ailments and conditions the industry claims it helps?

- Pineapples contain bromelien and manganese, believed to greatly reduce inflammation and swelling; they taste good too.

- Cross-training is just smart. Doing an activity other than your regular sport or art is beneficial for a variety of reasons. I think swimming, biking, yoga, martial arts, and soccer are among the best.

- Alternative medicine has always been around and is becoming more infused with convention practices. I personally cured a lifelong battle with a skin condition called eczema. At one point during my 20s, my eyelids would crack and bleed during outbreaks. I was even selected as a textbook study case by the University of Chicago medical school. Throughout my life, I was prescribed steroidal topical medications that have crappy side effects over prolonged periods of use. Later, I successfully found ways to permanently prevent outbreaks through diet and supplements such as sarsaparilla, yellow dock, and milk thistle. My skin is very healthy and heals quickly.

- I once watched my friend Mike Lowrie, who during a skate session repaired a huge gash with super glue. *WTF*. He had a one inch *very open* cut on his hand, went out to his car, cleaned the wound, glued it, and continued skating. There's no moral or advice in this story. It just blew my mind, mainly because it worked. I thought about the toxins that might enter his bloodstream but that was a few years ago and Mike is alive, living in New Mexico, and doing well. It was just a weird thing to see.

- Athlete Stoyan Angelov is a scientist dedicated to researching and the experimentation of innovative treatments to repair and regrow human tissue. That's a whole other book in itself—some very amazing stuff.

- On January 17, 2012, surfer/skateboarder Rex Flodstrom (page 199) was arrested after surfing at a Lake Michigan beach in Chicago. Although surfing is illegal at selected beaches, this was *not* one of them. He received several charges and a scheduled court date. Word spread quickly inside and out of the action sports community via news and social media prompting 11-time world champion Kelly

Slater to comment on the incident. Slater, in a most appropriate fashion, simply tweeted, "Surfing is not a crime." For the record, Rex's photo had been in *Tough Like You* a month before the incident. Also for the record, the outside temperature was in the 30's—nothing new to Rex. He has been winter surfing Lake Michigan for much of the last decade that we've been friends. Now that's tough.

- I've seriously considered writing a book on stretching in bed. Having developed a personal regimen of exercises, massage, and stretches before sleep as well as ones to do in the morning, I have found them to be extremely effective. The stretches noticeably help with healing, relaxation, awakening, and most certainly conditioning of the body. Self-massage has added benefits of helping to connect the body as a whole. I personally *want* to know what going on under my skin! Introducing your *own* fingers and hands to your feet, neck, scalp, knees, and overall muscular skeletal system is priceless. During a recent search of any like publication, I found that it had been done; someone has written a pamphlet on bed stretches and self-massage publications definitely exist. Crap! Maybe I'll just have to take it up a notch: "Super Stretches in Bed."

6

One day your life will flash before your eyes. Make
sure it's worth watching."
—Unknown

CONCLUSION

Tough Like You is the world's first piece of literature to combine
the experiences, advice, and expertise of action athletes and health
professionals, all on the subject of injuries, prevention,
conditioning, and longevity.

There are no conclusions; make your own. The very first sentence
of the foreword stated that this was *not* an answer book. Although
filled with useful information and real life testimony cover-to-
cover, it is only a guide. Better living comes from within, even if
inspired from the words of others.

A guide can only help you get to your destination. Ultimately, it's
you that must make the journey, so get to moving.

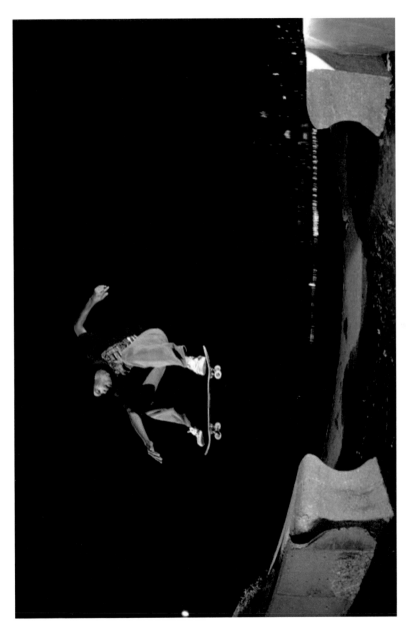

Timmy Johnson   Photo: Pat Shore

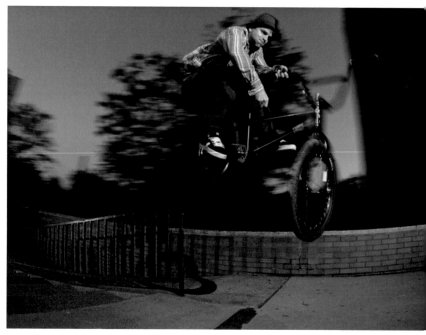

Brian Kachinsky   Photo: Davi

REFERENCES

Brian Tunney ESPN.com quote (2011) / Brian Kachinsky Intro

Focus East Coast Skate Magazine (2009 to 2011) Soap Box Columns

Racket Magazine (May 2008) / Silas Baxter-Neal Photo

Jesse Neuhaus quote courtesy of StreetCanoe.com

Airborne "Stand in the Door" (2011) Pike, Globalsecurity.org/military/ops/airborne

Dietician Section:

www.mayoclinic.com/health/water/NU00283

www.mayoclinic.com/health/dehydration/DS00561

www3.georgetown.edu/admin/auxiliarysrv/dining/Nutrition

www.heart.org/HEARTORG/Conditions/Cholesterol

www.mayoclinic.com/health/fat/NU00262/NSECTIONGROUP=2

www.michigantoday.umich.edu/2008/03/great-plate.php

Public Health Section:

Briggs, K. (July 7, 2009). SPORTS: 'Ramp It Up' www.americanindiannews.org/2009/07/sports-ramp-it-up-tells-story-of-native-americas-vibrant-skateboard-culture

Cash, R. E. (November, 2007). Dangerous High. Principal Leadership: Student Services, www.naspcenter.org/principals

Catalano, R. F., Berglund, M. L., Ryan, J. A. M., Lonczak, H. S., Hawkins, J. D. (2004). Positive Youth Development in the United States: Research Findings on Evaluations of Positive Youth Development Programs. *Annals of the American Academy of Political and Social Science*, 591, pp. 98-124

Centers for Disease Control and Prevention (CDC). (2003). Building a Healthier Future Through School Health Programs: Promising Practices in Chronic Disease Prevention and Control. A Public Health Framework for Action. *U.S. Department of Health and Human Services,* Chapter 9-1

Centers for Disease Control and Prevention (CDC). (2008). Guidelines for School Health Programs to Prevent Unintentional Injuries and Violence: Summary. *U.S. Department of Health and Human Services,* www.cdc.gov/HealthyYouth/injury/guidelines/summary.htm

Centers for Disease Control and Prevention (CDC). (2011). School Health Guidelines to Promote Healthy Eating and Physical Activity. *Morbidity and Mortality Weekly Report (MMWR), 60*(5), pp. 28-33

Healthwise. (2010). Emotional and Social Development, Ages 11 to 14 Years. University of Michigan C.S. Mott Children's Hospital, www.healthwise.org

Taliaferro, L. A., Rienzo, B. A., Miller, M. D., Pigg, R. M. Jr., Dodd, V. J. (2008). High school youth and suicide risk: exploring protection afforded through physical activity and sport participation. *Journal of School Health, 78*(10), pp. 545-53.

Thomson, L. (2009). How times have changed: Active transport literature review. *VicHealth, Website*: www.vichealth.vic.gov.au

Tony Hawk Foundation (2012). Why are skateparks beneficial to communities?

209 References

www.TonyHawkFoundation.org/faq

Glossary: Occasional source references using mayoclinic.com and University of Maryland Medical – umm.edu

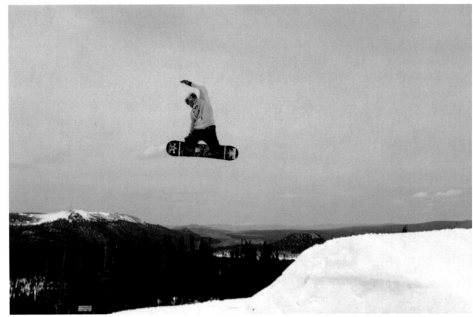

Ray Lang   Photo: Julian

ACKNOWLEDGMENTS

Thanks For The Support: Tough Like You Athletes & Health Consultants, Mat Hoffman, Tony Hawk, Character Skateboards, Focus East Coast Skate Magazine, Roseanne Segovia, 7G Consulting, LLC, Mendel College Prep Alumni Foundation, thuMp, Jess Bell and Windward Boardshop, Brain Kachinsky and Per Welinder for being more than helpful in connecting me to resources, Marci & Lawyers for the Creative Arts, Mom & Sis, Amos J Fuller Sr, Human Kinetics, Julian Bleecker & "Hello, Skater Girl", Odd Machine Productions-Chicago, DiggyPod Printing, Kickstarter, Thump the World Publishing, V.O.C, H.O.H. and V.A.C. Veteran Organizations, Autism Speaks, Captain Ed, Eric Sorensen & Laura Beth Nielsen, Joey Adamczyk, Jake Devries, Amy Limpinyakul, Krysle Ramos, Jeffrey Harvey, Eileen Mignoni, Greg Bell, Anthony Edward-Johnson, Javier Caballero, Danuta Godlewski, Artist P. Fuller, Fury Trucks, Stephanie Person, TC "The Crew", Spencer Montgomery, David Leep, Miriam Zmiewski-Angelova, Andrew Brady, Keisha Lackland, Ariel Ries, Antonio J. Martin, Susan Perry, Chris Raspante, Lee Larkins, Colin Commito, Larry LaMar, Al Butela, Ely Phillips, Joseph Linzemann, Jackson Hennessey, Azure Cadena, Mark Szymanski, Brandon Cole, Ryan Crane, Jimmy Smith III, Michael Owen, Patrick Shore, Shaolin Bez, Brad Piwko, Meleika E'non Gardner, Steve & Carla, Ryan-David Gray, Greg Ingram, Julian Izaguirre, Marfa Capodanno, Paul Zmiewski, Michael Enriquez-ZigZag, Emily Edelman, Rashad & Trent Malloy, Dorothy Perry, Ryan Vila, Marlène Jeffré, Jesus Arellanes, Greg Chapman, Corey Henderson, Coleman Sdrawde, Korie Leigh, Alexander Fuller, Timeless Classic, Shawn Turner, Bill and Cream City, Zoe Pope, Stephanie & Esmeralda, Matt Frankland, Elena & Ariel Rubin, Temper, Bill Natale at I.C.B, Wilson Warriors, all Chicago and skater owned shops everywhere.

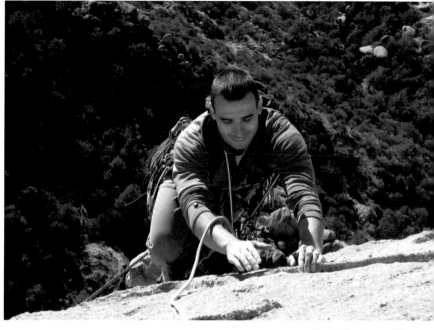

Photo: Courtesy of Stoyan

INDEX

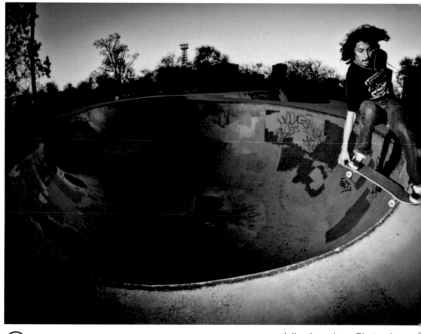

GLOSSARY

Julian Izaguirre   Photo: Jesus A

100 Percent the state of being basically injury free and able to fully perform

Accidents mishaps, collisions, unexpected loss of control

ACL anterior cruciate ligament. One of the four major ligaments of the human knee

ACL Reconstruction surgery to rebuild the ligament with a new ligament

Action Athletes athletes that partake in non-conventional sports and activities often with higher risk of injury

Action Sports activities having a higher level of inherent danger often involving speed, stunts, height, and a high level of physical exertion

Acupuncture treats patients by insertion and manipulation of thin needles in the body to regulate the flow of an energy-like entity called *qi*. Acupuncture aims to correct imbalances in the flow of qi by stimulation of anatomical locations on or under the skin called points

Acupuncturist physicians who practice acupuncture

Acute extremely great or serious

Addiction physical or psychological dependency to an external stimuli

Adrenal Glands also known as suprarenal glands, are endocrine glands that are chiefly responsible for releasing hormones in response to stress through the synthesis of corticosteroids such as cortisol

Adrenaline also known as epinephrine. Adrenaline is a hormone and a neurotransmitter. It increases heart rate, constricts blood vessels, dilates air passages and participates in the fight-or-flight response. A hormone produced in your body that arises in dire circumstances. Adrenaline has allowed a normal mom to lift a car and save her baby

Adrenaline Junky one who feeds off adrenaline and uses it to push themselves in sports, life, or crime

Airborne a subdivision of the Armed Forces that specializes in combat parachuting

Amateur an individual that is recognized for their talents but not yet paid

Amped the mental state of being "fired up" and ready to perform

Analgesics a drug or medicine given to reduce pain without resulting in loss of consciousness

Anatomy the science that studies the structure of the body

Anti-inflammatory Drugs/NSAIDs medications used primarily to treat inflammation, mild to moderate pain, and fever

Antioxidants substances that may protect cells from the damage caused by unstable molecules known as free radicals

Arthroscopic/Arthroscopic a procedure that uses a tube-like device to examine, diagnose and treat a joint (knee, hip, wrist, shoulder, ankle, etc.)

Autonomic controlled by the autonomic nervous system, acts involuntarily

Bails attempts to get away from a missed or purposely ditched trick

Blunt slides a skateboard trick where the tail of a skateboard slides on the rail or ledge and the rest of the skateboard is above the rail or ledge

Blunt Trauma non-penetrating trauma caused to a body part, either by impact, injury or physical attack

BMX Bicycle motocross

Bodywork a term used in alternative medicine to describe any therapeutic or personal development technique that involves working with the human body in a form involving manipulative therapy, breath work, or energy medicine

Bromelien an extract from the stems of pineapples. As a supplement it is thought to have anti-inflammatory properties

Bursitis inflammation of the fluid-filled sac (bursa) that lies between a tendon and skin, or between a tendon and bone

Calcium the most abundant mineral in the body, it is found in some foods, added to others, and is available as a dietary supplement and present in some medicines

Carbohydrates a component of food classified as simple or complex. They are the most important source of energy for your body

Cardio Fitness light-to-moderate intensity activities performed for extended periods of time to help strengthen heart and circulation health

CAT Scan Computerized Axial Tomography. A procedure that assists in diagnosing tumors, fractures, bony structures, and infections in the body

Catabolism degradative metabolism involving the release of energy and resulting in the breakdown of complex materials (as proteins or lipids) within the body

Chinese Medicine a broad range of medicine practices sharing common theoretical concepts developed in China and based on a tradition of more than 2,000 years, including various forms of herbal medicine, acupuncture, massage, exercise (qigong), and dietary therapy

Cholesterol a fat (lipid) produced by the liver and is crucial for normal body functioning

Christ Air invented by skater Christian Hosoi, an aerial skateboarding trick where, while flying in the air, the skateboarder picks up his board into one of his hands and then spreads his arms and straightens his legs forming a pose that resembles Jesus Christ on the cross

Chronic a disease or other health condition that is persistent or long-lasting

Circadian Rhythm is an internal biological clock that regulates a variety of biological processes according to an approximate 24-hour period. Mostly associated with our sleep patterns

Collagen Fibers mostly found in fibrous tissues such as tendon, ligament and skin, and is also abundant in cornea, cartilage, bone, blood vessels, the gut, and intervertebral disc

Complex Carb often referred to as starch or starches. They are found naturally in foods and also abundantly refined in processed foods

Concussion a type of traumatic brain injury that is caused by a blow to the head or body, a fall, or another injury that jars or shakes the brain inside the skull

Condition state of, or diagnosis related to, health or wellness

Contrast Therapy the effective use of heat and cold as an injury healing technique

Contusion a bruise, of relatively minor hematoma of tissue, in which capillaries and sometimes venules are damaged by trauma

Core refers to the body minus the legs and arms. Functional movements are highly dependent on the core

Cortisol a chemical hormone produced by your body to manage stress. The stress can be physical, mental and emotional

Cramp unpleasant, often painful sensations caused by muscle contraction or over shortening

Cross-training refers to an athlete training in sports other than their usual, with a goal of improving overall performance

Degenerative is a disease or condition in which the function or structure of the affected tissues or organs will progressively deteriorate over time

Dehydration means your body does not have as much water and fluids as it should

Deltoid Ligament is a strong, flat, triangular band, attached to the apex and anterior and posterior borders of the medial malleolus

Dexterity physical movement, especially in the use of the hands

Diabetes a lifelong (chronic) disease in which there are high levels of sugar in the blood

Diet the kinds of food that a person eats

Dietitian a person that supervises the preparation and service of food, develops modified diets, participates in research, and educates individuals and groups on good nutrition

Discs lie between adjacent vertebrae in the spine. Each disc forms a cartilaginous joint to allow slight movement of the vertebrae, and acts as a ligament to hold the vertebrae together

DIY Do It Yourself

DNA a nucleic acid containing the genetic instructions used in the development and functioning of all known living organisms

Dysbiosis refers to a condition with microbial imbalances on or within the body

Ectomorph characterized by long and thin muscles/limbs and low fat storage; usually referred to as slim

EFAs contains the essential fatty acids that we must obtain through our diet because they cannot be made by our bodies

Endurance Training exercising to increase stamina and endurance

Epidemic a rapid spread or increase in the occurrence of something

Epidurals steroid injections can temporarily relieve many forms of low back pain and leg pain (sciatica) and help a patient progress with rehab and exercise

Epsom Salt (Magnesium Sulfate Heptahydrate) is a well known product used in bath salts for softening the skin and relaxing sore muscles

Essential Amino Acids are those that are necessary for good health but cannot be synthesized by the body and so must be found in diet

Estrogen refers to a group of chemically similar compounds or hormones that play a pivotal role in the development of female sexual traits and characteristics

Evil Knievel an American daredevil and entertainer. In his career, he attempted over 75 ramp-to-ramp motorcycle jumps between 1965 and 1980. The 433 broken bones he suffered during his career earned an entry in the Guinness Book of World Records as the survivor of "most bones broken in a lifetime"

Exercise Physiology the study of the acute responses and chronic adaptations to a wide-range of physical exercise conditions

Falls loss of control with full contact to ground or object being performed on

Fascia a layer of fibrous tissue that permeates the human body. A fascia is a connective tissue that surrounds muscles, groups of muscles, blood vessels, and nerves

Fish Oil is oil derived from the tissues of oily fish. Fish oils contain omega-3 fatty acids

Flavonoids anti-oxidants found naturally in plants

Flax Seed Oil comes from the seeds of the flax plant and contains both omega-3 and omega-6 fatty acids

Foodist a person whose diet consists mainly of raw foods

Fracture a break in the continuity of the bone

Frontside Crook a grind on a skateboard where the skater is facing the rail or ledge when he pops and grinds front truck and the nose pointed toward the grind rail

Globulin Hormones sex steroid-binding globulin (SSBG) is a glycoprotein that binds to sex hormones, testosterone, and estradiol

Gluconeogenesis the synthesis of glucose from molecules that are not carbohydrates, such as amino and fatty acids

Glucosamine a natural compound that is found in healthy cartilage

Glucose a carbohydrate, and is the most important simple sugar in human metabolism

Glycation a process where sugar and protein molecules combine to form a tangled mess of tissue

Goal-oriented to work towards a specific task completion or level of achievement

Grind mainly a skateboard maneuver where the metal of the trucks ride a surface without use of the wheels

Half-pipe a ramp used for action sports in the shape of a half circle

Hammer slang for an amazing or difficult trick

Handlebar Spin a bike trick where the handle bars are spun around while airborne

Hard Flip a skateboard trick that combines a frontside pop shove-it with a kick-flip

Head Protection gear worn in action sports and other activities to reduce risk of head injury

Healing restoration of damaged living tissue, organs and biological system to normal function

Health the level of functional or metabolic efficiency of a living being. It is the general condition of a person's mind, body and spirit, usually meaning to be free from illness, injury or pain. In many action sports "healthy" is the ability to perform regardless of what an individual's actual condition may be

Health Consultant a guide who provides information and advice for a person's health and wellness

Health Professionals highly skilled workers, in professions that usually require extensive knowledge of their area of health care

Herbal Medicine also called botanical medicine or phytomedicine— refers to using a plant's seeds, berries, roots, leaves, bark, or flowers for medicinal purposes. Herbalism has a long tradition of use outside of conventional medicine

Hernia occurs when part of an internal organ bulges through a weak area of muscle

Hipper slang term for a bruised hip usually caused from a slam

Hobbyist a person who practices an activity solely for recreation

Holistic a concept in medical practice upholding that all aspects of people's needs, psychological, physical and social should be taken into account and seen as a whole

Homies street term for individuals that hang together often

Hormones a chemical released by a cell or a gland in one part of the body that sends out messages that affect cells in other parts

Hydration the supply and retention of adequate water in our bodies

Hypoglycemic abnormally diminished content of glucose in the blood

Ice Climbing Crampon spiked devices clamped to an ice climbers boots. The front spikes poke straight out and are often kicked into the ice allowing them to gain footing

Immune System a system of biological structures and processes within an organism that protects against disease

Impact to make contact with, in action sports, usually forcefully or high impact

Industry the business end of action sports—companies, events, contest, media

Inflammation the basic way our bodies reacts to infection, irritation or other injury, the key feature being redness, warmth, swelling, and pain

Injury damage to your body

Inner child the child-like side within each of us that is ultimately creative, alive, energetic, and simplified

Jake Brown Australian professional skateboarder that made world news after a 45 foot fall during the 2007 X Games that he eventually walked away from with injuries

Jeet Kune Do a hybrid martial arts system and life philosophy founded by martial artist Bruce Lee

John Cardiel a legendary professional skateboarder injured in 2003 from a non-skating accident and told he would never walk again. After five months of rehabilitation in the hospital and a few months in a wheelchair, he was able to regain the use of his legs and remains an active figure in the world of skateboarding as well as cycling

Kinesiology also known as human kinetics, it is the scientific study of human movement

Laser Heel Flip frontside 360 heel-flip but the board spins behind you. Opposite of tre-flip, opposite flip, opposite spin

Lateral Deltoid the muscle forming the rounded contour of the shoulder

Lateral Meniscus crescent-shaped bands of thick, rubbery cartilage attached to the shinbone

Legend a very well known, usually highly respected person

Leptin a protein hormone that plays a key role in regulating energy intake and energy expenditure, including appetite and metabolism

Ligament fibrous tissue that connects bones to other bones and supports organs

Lines the path that skateboarders, bikers, snowboarders and other action athletes take while doing a run of tricks

Lip The edge of ramp, bowl, pool or ledge usually used to grind or other tricks

Longevity a long duration of health, performance and productivity

Lumbar the largest segments of the movable part of the vertebral column

M.E.A.T. stands for Movement, Exercise, Analgesics, and Treatments

Magnesium plays important roles in the structure and the function of the human body. The adult human body contains about 25 grams of magnesium

Manganese a trace mineral that is present in tiny amounts in the body. It is found mostly in bones, the liver, kidneys, and pancreas

Martial Arts extensive systems of technical practices and traditions of combat that are practiced for a variety of reasons

Massage the working of other tissue and deeper layers of muscle and connective tissue using various techniques for various purposes, to enhance function, aid in healing, promote relaxation and well-being

Mat Hoffman legendary BMX rider with a history of several injuries and miraculous recoveries

Mayo Clinic a not-for-profit medical practice and medical research group specializing in treating difficult patients

MCL one of the four major ligaments of the knee

Medial Meniscus situated in the knee joint plays the role of a load bearer, shock absorber, knee stabilizer, etc.

Medical Marijuana refers to the use of the herb cannabis as medicine or herbal therapy

MegaRamp a very large ramp structure designed by professional Skateboarder Danny Way, unveiled in 2002

Melatonin a hormone secreted by the pineal gland in the brain. It helps regulate other hormones and maintains the body's circadian rhythm, or sleep cycle

Mental Visualization a mental routine or exercise that improves one's efficiency when actually physically performing the activity. The same areas of the brain are activated whether you are thinking about the activity or actually doing it

Metabolism refers to all the physical and chemical processes in the body that convert or use energy

Mono, Poly and Unsaturated Fats organic compounds that are made up of carbon, hydrogen, and oxygen. They are a source of energy in foods

Motor-unit Recruitment the progressive activation of a muscle by successive recruitment of contractile units (motor units) to accomplish increasing gradations of contracting strength

MRI magnetic resonance imaging (MRI) is a test that uses a magnetic field and pulses of radio wave energy to make pictures of organs and structures inside the body

MSM methylsulfonylmethane (MSM) is an organosulfur compound used as a supplement to relieve pain and inflammation

Muscle is a contractile tissue. Muscle cells contain contractile filaments that move past each other and change the size of the cell. They are classified as skeletal, cardiac, or smooth muscles. Their function is to produce force and cause motion. We have more than 600 muscles in our bodies

Muscle Memory movement that muscles gradually become familiar with

Musculature the system or arrangement of muscles in a body, a part of the body, or an organ

Musculoskeletal the system of muscles, tendons, ligaments, bones, joints and associated tissues that move the body and maintain its form

Narcotics a wide variety of substances that dulled the senses and relieve pain

Non-Union Break a bone fracture that does not heal itself without the use of surgical implants

Nutrient a chemical needed to live and grow or a substance used in metabolism which must be taken in from a source of nourishment, especially a nourishing ingredient in a food

Nutrition materials necessary (in the form of food) to support life

Omega-3 fatty acids considered essential that are necessary for human health but the body can't produce. You have to get them through food

Orthopedist a physician that specializes in the prevention or correction of injuries or disorders of the skeletal system and associated muscles, joints, and ligaments

Osteoarthritis the most common form of arthritis. It causes pain, swelling and reduced motion in your joints

Pain Killers any member of the group of drugs used to relieve pain

Patella a flat, triangular bone located at the front of the knee joint. Also called the kneecap

Pharmaceutical chemical substance intended for use in the medical diagnosis, cure, treatment, or prevention of injury and illness

Physical Therapy a branch of rehabilitative medicine aimed at helping patients maintain, recover or improve their physical abilities

Physiotherapy another name for Physical Therapy

Posture the position in which you hold your body upright against gravity while standing, sitting or lying down

Potassium a very important mineral for the proper function of all cells, tissues, and organs in the human body especially the heart, kidneys, muscles, nerves, and digestive system

Primo is when a skateboarder's board lands on its side unintentionally or purposefully

Professional a person who is paid to undergo a specialized set of tasks and to complete them for a fee. Following an occupation as a means of livelihood or for gain

Protective Gear clothing, padding, helmet, etc. that protect one's body during an activity

Protein the building blocks of life. The body needs protein to repair and maintain itself

Proximal interphalangeal (PIP) Joints the finger joint closest to the knuckle

R.I.C.E. stands for Rest, Ice, Compression and Elevation

Recovery return to a normal condition

Recuperate recover from injury, illness or exertion

Rehabilitation restore to good condition, operation or make healthy again

Resiliency the ability to spring back from and successfully adapt to adversity, injury, etc.

Rip / Rippin slang term used for when an action athlete is committed and performing hard

Rock Climbing a physically and mentally demanding sport where large rock formations are scaled

Rolled ankle athletic term for a sprained ankle

Rotator cuff the group of muscles and their tendons that act to stabilize the shoulder

Ruptured discs a common back condition that leads to irritation of spinal nerves and can cause back and leg pain

Sciatic Nerve is the largest and longest nerve in the body

Scoliosis a medical condition in which a person's spine is curved from side to side

Scoped a small, thin arthroscope gives knee surgeons clear view to look inside your knee and repair damage and tears

Self-healing the process of recovery motivated by and directed by the injured person themselves

Self-help implementing practices or educating yourself to better yourself

Serotonin a neurotransmitter, involved in the transmission of nerve impulses

Skateboarding active pursuit and involvement in riding a skateboard

SkunkBelly childhood contact skateboard game played by author

Slam a really hard fall, sometimes resulting in injury

Soma the "ideal pleasure drug" that kept society from feeling pain or unhappiness in novel *Brave New World* by Aldous Huxley

Sports Drink common drinks that hydrate and replenish electrolytes

Sports Medicine deals with physical fitness, treatment and prevention of injuries related to sports and exercise

Sprain an injury to a ligament caused by excessive stretching. The ligament can have a partial tear, or it can be completely torn apart

Starches the most common carbohydrate in the human diet and is contained in many staple foods

Stoked excited about something presently happening or anticipated to happen

Straight edge someone who refrains from using alcohol, tobacco, and other recreational drugs

Street a term used in action sports to define location or style. Street is derived from performing in areas not designed for the specific activity

Stretch a form of exercise or a pre-exercise sometimes called warming up to prepare body for specific activity

Sub-acute a medical problem that is not exactly acute or chronic, rather somewhere in between

Suicidality the likelihood of an individual completing suicide

Surfing the sport or art which involves riding water and waves on a board

Swellbow a common word to describe an action sports injury to the elbow or forearm area

Systemic is one that affects a number of organs and tissues, or affects the body as a whole

Tendon tough band of fibrous connective tissue that usually connects muscle to bone and is capable of withstanding tension

Tendonitis occurs when there is inflammation of tendons

Testosterone a steroid hormone from the androgen group. Primarily secreted in the testes of males and the ovaries of females. It is the principal male sex hormone

The Great Plate a diagram created by the University of Michigan illustrating essential food groups to help people build healthy meals

Therapy is process of or attempt to improve or cure a health problem, usually following a diagnosis

Thrasher legendary skateboard magazine and also a term to refer to one that skates or surfs fast, agile and committed

Thyroid thyroid gland controls how quickly the body uses energy, makes proteins, and controls how sensitive the body is to other hormones

Titanium Joint newer joint replacement technology using the alloy titanium

Tricks specialized maneuvers done while performing action sports

Triglycerides a type of fat found in your blood. Your body uses them for energy. You need some triglycerides for good health. But high triglycerides can raise your risk of heart disease

Tuck & Roll assuming the fetal position mid-bail to minimize bodily damage

Tweak to sprain, injure or in general hurt an area of the body

Ulna one of the two long bones in the forearm

Unprocessed Foods food eaten in their raw, natural state

Vegetarian the practice of following plant-based diets (fruits, vegetables, etc.), with or without the inclusion of dairy products or eggs, and with the exclusion of meat, red meat, poultry, and seafood

Vert the part of a ramp, wall or other obstacle with no curvature, straight vertical

Vitruvian Man a world-renowned drawing of the human figure created by Leonardo da Vinci

Wellness the state of, or proactive pursuit of health physically, emotionally and mentally

X Games annual action sports competition event. The inaugural X Games was held in the summer of 1995 in Rhode Island

Yoga a physical, mental, and spiritual discipline, originating in ancient India

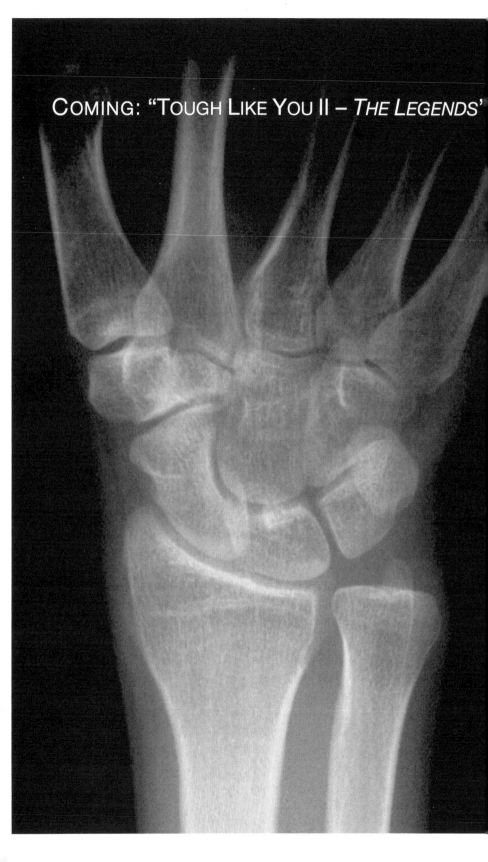
COMING: "TOUGH LIKE YOU II – *THE LEGENDS*"